The AGP System

Manual for the Documentation
of Psychopathology
in Gerontopsychiatry

Edited and Translated from the German
by William Guy and Thomas A. Ban

In Collaboration with
John Hoenig, Siegfried Kanowski,
V. A. Kral, Alice Leeds, and Jan Libiger

Springer-Verlag
Berlin Heidelberg New York Tokyo

William Guy, Ph. D.
Associate Professor of Psychiatry

Thomas A. Ban, M. D.
Professor of Psychiatry

Vanderbilt University, 242 Medical Arts Building,
1211 21st Avenue, South Nashville, TN 37212, USA

ISBN-13:978-3-540-15440-2 e-ISBN-13:978-3-642-82514-9
DOI: 10.1007/978-3-642-82514-9

Library of Congress Cataloging in Publication Data. Main entry under title:
The AGP system. Bibliography: p. Includes index. 1. AGP System. I. Guy, William.
II. Ban, Thomas A. RC451.4.A5A38 1985 618.97'689'075 85-14837

2125/3140-543210

Foreword

Among the more frequently quoted epidemiological facts in current public health discussions are: (a) the elderly today represent about 10% of the population of the industrialized world; (b) the third world nations are moving in the same direction; (c) the trend toward a growing proportion of the aged in the world population will continue over the next few decades; (d) people over 80 now represent the fastest growing sector in North America; (e) in the elderly, general morbidity – and particularly morbidity of the central nervous system – is many times that in the younger population; (f) 5% of those over 65 years of age and 20% of those over 80 suffer from some degree of dementia. A global tidal wave of patients suffering from Alzheimer's disease (or senile dementia) is threatening to engulf us by the year 2000.

This disease, which is, at our present state of knowledge, irreversible, and other age-related dementias are perhaps the most sinister forms of any disability. They deprive their victims not only of their physical capacities but also of their autonomy and their ability to think and to make decisions for themselves. The future cost of psychogeriatric diseases in terms of suffering for individuals, stress for families, demand for manpower, and budgetary requirements for governments could become astronomical.

What can be done to counter this awesome threat? We do not know the causes of the most common dementias nor do we have any effective treatments to prevent these diseases. The only hope lies in gerontological and geriatric research. But no research is possible without a body of systematically collected, reliable data. Here we find one of the reasons for the gaps in our gerontopsychiatric knowledge: our methods for gathering descriptive and psychopathological data from geriatric patients are poorly developed. They are, in fact, almost primitive when compared with the quite sophisticated methods available for similar purposes in other areas of modern psychiatry.

Why did we allow this anachronistic state of affairs to develop? Probably for the same reasons that may explain the following strange paradox. We know much more about the morbid pathology and pathophysiology of organic brain syndromes than about the so-called functional disorders, the neuroses and psychoses, yet we have fewer effective treatments for the organic than for the functional disorders. This is almost certainly a consequence of the fundamental doctrine that destroyed neurons do not regenerate – and the belief that we are thus condemned to therapeutic nihilism in all organic brain disorders, including most gerontopsychiatric diseases.

We now know that this is not true, because organic brain diseases do not destroy neurons all at once. Before a neuron is destroyed it usually passes through stages of impaired metabolism and compromised functioning during which the damage is still reversible. However, if we want to do research on therapeutic interventions that might reverse such damage and delay or prevent the development of a finally irreversible brain disorder, we must first be able to recognize its early manifestations, that is, diagnose accurately and reliably its early symptoms.

The lack of adequate methods for gathering and documenting data in gerontopsychiatry constitutes a major barrier to basic and clinical research. How can we investigate the early stages of organic brain disease if we can recognize it with certainty only in its advanced stages? How can we conduct clinical trials with potentially therapeutic agents if we, for example, cannot even distinguish the manifestations of normal aging from early symptoms of Alzheimer's disease?

If we want to tackle these problems in an orderly fashion we will have to go back to the grass roots of all clinical knowledge – the clinical phenomena. Long ago, medicine, having freed itself from magic and superstition, created its base on the clinical observation of phenomena, signs, and symptoms. This led to the articulation of clinical syndromes and, eventually, to the formulation of nosological concepts. Nosological concepts, in turn, gave rise to hypotheses and theories about the structural, pathophysiological, and psychopathological substrates of these concepts.

Unfortunately, psychiatry is a disadvantaged discipline in regard to diagnosis because, in contrast to other medical disciplines, it has practically no objective diagnostic criteria at its disposal, at least no external criteria that have the objective equivalence of meter readings. Most psychiatric observations and, implicitly, diagnoses are based on behavioral phenomena which involve a subjective component in both the subject and the observer. For the subject, this subjectivity rests in self-awareness and emotionality, while for the observer it lies in perceiving, interpreting, and rating behavioral phenomena. As long as we do not possess reliable biological markers, it is mandatory that refined, non-physical diagnostic instruments such as structured interviews, rating scales, assessment inventories, and operationally defined descriptions be developed. Validated and standardized for optimal interrater and intertest reliability, such diagnostic instruments can supply a high degree of objectivity.

Several such diagnostic instruments have been developed and have proved their value for clinical management and research in adult psychiatry. However, there has been a conspicuous paucity of equally sophisticated and comprehensive diagnostic instruments in gerontopsychiatry. The consequent lack of precise and reliable diagnostic data has inhibited clinical research and progress in the field. Gerontopsychiatry acquires a special complexity owing to the fact that, in addition to the emergence of specific psychiatric diseases that are characteristic only for the aged, there are also interactions between other, more general psychiatric disorders and the normal aging process which may change the usual symptomatic expression of these disorders.

The present Manual is divided into three major sections containing six Assessment Documents, detailed instructions for raters and a well-organized glossary. An appendix provides valuable lists of psychopathological symptoms and somatic signs in both English and German. References and a well-prepared index are other useful parts of the Manual that can facilitate subsequent computer processing of the encoded assessment sheets which document demographic data, psychiatric history, psychopathological symptoms, somatic signs, and diagnoses.

The publication of this Manual will go a long way toward closing the disturbing gap in the systematic approach to phenomenology, psychopathology, and diagnosis in gerontopsychiatry that has long existed. The Manual has been developed over a period of almost 10 years through painstaking work at four major universities in Germany, Switzerland, and the United States. It is difficult to think of any better guarantee of the relevance and authenticity of the system.

H. E. Lehmann, M.D.
Professor Emeritus
Department of Psychiatry
McGill University
Montreal, Quebec, Canada

Contents

Introduction

AGP stands for *Arbeitsgemeinschaft für Gerontopsychiatrie,* or Association for Gerontopsychiatry. This association of German-speaking psychiatric professionals developed the assessment and documentation system which bears the name "the AGP system."

The first version of AGP system was developed by the Gerontopsychiatric Division of the Free University of Berlin and the Psychiatric Clinic of the University of Lausanne in consultation with the Psychiatric Clinic of the University of Freiburg during the early and middle 1970s [1, 6, 8, 9, 10, 11, 14, 16]. To a large extent, this version was deliberately structured to be compatible with the AMP-II system designed for the assessment of psychopathology in the adult population.

In 1978, Jan Libiger, then a WHO Fellow in Biological Psychiatry at the Tennessee Neuropsychiatric Institute, and T. A. Ban produced the initial English translation of the first version of the AGP. At the same time, an English translation of the AMP-II was in progress at Nashville. Efforts were directed at making the two translations as compatible as possible so that a commonality of assessment across the life span would be enhanced.

As this work was nearing completion, a new revision of the present system, AMDP-III, was published in Germany. Since it superseded the previous version, an entirely new translation of AMDP-III was then undertaken by W. Guy and T. A. Ban – a translation published in 1982 [13]. Little progress was made with the English AGP until 1981, when a new German version based upon the AMDP-III was received from S. Kanowski. An entirely new translation of the AGP, incorporating large segments of the new AMDP, was then prepared. This translation was then reviewed by our collaborators, S. Kanowski, A. Leeds, J. Hoenig, and V. A. Kral, whose painstaking examination and insightful criticisms of the text have resulted in the present version. Finally we wish to express our gratitude to Mildred Harrington for her skill in typing the manuscript and her patience with the authors.

W. Guy and T. A. Ban

Documentation

The AGP system consists of six integrated parts:

Part 1 – Anamnesis – Demographic Data. This section consists of two pages and contains 24 items describing the patient's personal, marital, residential, educational, and occupational status at the time of the examination.

Part 2 – Anamnesis – Psychiatric History. This section consists of two pages and contains 12 additional items dealing primarily with the psychiatric history of the patient and his family, prior treatment, and a description of the present episode.

Part 3 – Psychopathological Symptoms. This section consists of a single page and contains 107 items, most of which have been derived from the AMDP-III and which focus upon general psychopathology.

Part 4 – Psychopathological Symptoms. This section consists of a single page and contains an additional 69 symptoms which focus assessment on the symptomatology of the psychoorganic syndrome.

Part 5 – Somatic Signs. This section consists of a single page and contains 76 items which assess somatic signs of conditions prevalent in geriatric patients. Many of the AMDP-III symptoms which may be consequences of drug treatment and/or psychopathology are included here.

Part 6 – Diagnoses. This section consists of a single page and contains space for the encoding of three psychiatric and four somatic diagnoses as well as estimates of certitude regarding the diagnosis and the age of first manifestation.

All of the AGP documentation sheets are designed to serve as both encoding and transcribing vehicles. While all six Parts can be encoded directly, only Parts 3, 4, and 5 can be transcribed directly to cards, tape, and entered into the computer without recoding. Parts 1, 2, and 6 require some numeric recoding prior to transcription.

Plans for North American Processing

The Tennessee Neuropsychiatric Institute version of the Biometric Laboratory Information Processing System (BLIPS-TNI) has been programmed for the processing and analysis of the English AMDP-III system. Given their commonality in design and format, it is planned to develop a similar capability for the AGP system.

Briefly, BLIPS is a modularly constructed integrated series of computer programs which produce documentation for a variety of scientific data inputs [12]. It was developed at George Washington University under the auspices of the National Institute of Mental Health as part of the Early Clinical Drug Evaluation Program (ECDEU) of the Psychopharmacology Research Branch. BLIPS was designed to process all types of assessment data and, therefore, the insertion of data from the AGP system can be accomplished without extensive reprogramming. After entry into the computer in the form of a work file, four levels of editing are utilized to produce "clean data." Once accomplished, a master file is created for subsequent analytic procedures. BLIPS-TNI has an extensive catalog of statistical procedures which can be selected for specific use as well as a series of standard data outputs which provide a variety of descriptive displays for the interpretation of statistical findings.

AGP Part 1. Demographic Data

CLINIC/HO. ____ STUDY______ RATER______ DATE EXAM____/____/____
M D Y

PT INITIALS______ PT. NO._____ PERIOD_____

STATUS IN___ OUT___ PART___ OTH__________

SEX M__ F__ RACE W__ B__ I__ O__ OTH_____ __________

BIRTHDATE ____/____/____
M D Y

---

1. SOURCE: Primary_____ Secondary____ Both____ NA____
2. AGE:______ NA______
3. MARITAL STATUS: Single__ Mar'd__ Sep'd__ Div.__ Widw__ Cohab__ NA__
4. NATIONALITY: Citizen by birth___ Naturalized___ Alien___ Stateless___ NA___
5. CHILDREN: A. Number: 0___ 1___ 2___ 3___ 4___ 5___ >5___ NA___
   B. Presently Living: 0___ 1___ 2___ 3___ 4___ 5___ >5___ NA__
6. SIBLINGS: A. Number: 0___ 1___ 2___ 3___ 4___ 5___ >5___ NA__
   B. Presently Living: 0___ 1___ 2___ 3___ 4___ 5___ >5___ NA__
   C. Twin: Y____ N____ NA____
7. RELIGION: Protestant___ Roman Catholic___ Hebrew___ None___
   Other (Specify) ____________________ NA_____
8. RELIGIOUS CONVICTION: Weak___ Average___ Strong___ NA___

AGP Part 1. Demographic Data *(continued)*

9. TRUSTEESHIP: Y___ N___ NA___

10. GUARDIANSHIP: Y___ N___ NA___

11. RESIDENTIAL SETTING: Urban___ Suburban___ Rural___ NA___

12. RESIDENTIAL STATUS: A. Present residence: Own Home___ Rental Accom.___
Subtenant___ Indep. geriatric___ Supervised geriatric___ Nursing home___
General/psychiatric hosp.___ No Fixed Address___ Other___ NA___
B. Institutional residence: Pat.___ Spouse___ Pt/Spouse___ NA___

13. HOUSEHOLD COMPOSITION (excluding pt): Spouse___ Children___ Siblings___
Parents___ Grandchildren___ Other___ NA___

14. HOUSEHOLD INCOME STATUS: A. Level: Dependent___ Marginal___ Adequate___ NA___
B. Income Source: Pension___ Salary___ Capital Assets___
Social Agency___ Other___ NA___
C. Number Supported by Income: 1___ 2___ 3___ 4___ 5___ >5___ NA___

15. EDUCATION:

	Completed	Partial	NA
Special Education	___	___	___
Elementary (1-8)	___	___	___
High School (9-12)	___	___	___
College	___	___	___
Graduate School	___	___	___
NA	___	___	___

16. VOCATIONAL TRAINING:

	Completed	Partial	NA
Apprenticeship	___	___	___
Business/Technical School	___	___	___
Other: ___	___	___	___

17. OCCUPATION

A. Level

	Patient		Spouse	
	Highest Attained	Last Job	Highest Attained	Last Job
Homemaker	___	___	___	___
Homemaker-2nd job	___	___	___	___
Student	___	___	___	___
Self-employed Worker	___	___	___	___
Self-employed Entrepreneur	___	___	___	___
Major Professional	___	___	___	___
Minor Professional	___	___	___	___
Skilled Worker	___	___	___	___
Semiskilled Worker	___	___	___	___
Unskilled Worker	___	___	___	___
NA	___	___	___	___

B. Presently unemployed: Y___ N___ NA___

18. RETIREMENT: A. Not retired___ Retired usual___ early___ late___ NA___

B. Voluntary___ Involuntary___ No job___ NA___

AGP Part 1. Demographic Data *(continued)*

19. FREETIME ACTIVITIES: Y___ N___ NA___

20. SOCIAL RELATIONSHIPS:

    A. Objective: Frequent___ Seldom___ None___ NA___

    B. Subjective: Satisfying___ Unsatisfying___ NA___

21. PREVIOUS CARE: None___ Spouse___ Family___ Friend___
    Charitable Religious Agency___ Health Facility___ Other Gov/t Agency___
    Other (specify)______________________________ NA___

22. REFERRAL SOURCE: Self___ Spouse/Family___ Physician___ Clinic/hosp___
    Service Agency___ Other (specify)______________________ NA___

23. TYPE OF ADMISSION: Voluntary___ Involuntary___ NA___

24. REASON FOR ADMISSION: Suicidal attempt___ Dangerous/self___
    Dangerous/others___ Other (specify)______________________ NA___

AGP Part 2. Psychiatric History

CLINIC/HOSP_____ STUDY_____ RATER_____ DATE EXAM____/____/____
M D Y

PT. INITIALS_____ PT. NO._____ PERIOD_____

STATUS IN___ OUT___ PART___ OTH__________

SEX M__ F__ RACE W__ B__ I__ O__ OTH____________________

BIRTHDATE____/____/____
M D Y

---

25. FAMILY PSYCHIATRIC HISTORY:

A. 1st Degree Relatives: None___ Suspected___ Confirmed___ Hosp.___ NA___

B. Distant Relatives: None___ Suspected___ Confirmed___ Hosp.___ NA___

26. PREVIOUS NON-PSYCHIATRIC ILLNESS: No CNS___ Oth Org___ Diseases NA___

A. CNS Diseases	None	Suspected	Confirmed	Sequelae	NA	B. Other Organic	None	Suspected	Confirmed	Sequelae	NA
Inflammatory	_	_	_	_	_	Inflammatory	_	_	_	_	_
Trauma	_	_	_	_	_	Trauma	_	_	_	_	_
Tumor	_	_	_	_	_	Tumor	_	_	_	_	_
Constitutional	_	_	_	_	_	Constitutional	_	_	_	_	_
Intoxication	_	_	_	_	_	Intoxication	_	_	_	_	_
Epilepsy	_	_	_	_	_	Metabclic	_	_	_	_	_
Surgical	_	_	_	_	_	Cardicvascular	_	_	_	_	_

AGP Part 2. Psychiatric History *(continued)*

27. PREVIOUS PSYCHIATRIC ILLNESS:

None___	None	Suspected	Confirmed	Sequelae	NA
Constitutional/ childhood illness	___	___	___	___	___
Endogenous illness	___	___	___	___	___
Exogenous illness	___	___	___	___	___
Psychoneurotic reactions	___	___	___	___	___
Addiction	___	___	___	___	___

Alcohol___ Hypnotic/analgesic___ Opiate___ Other___ **NA**___

28. NUMBER OF PREVIOUS PSYCHIATRIC ADMISSIONS:

0___ 1___ 2___ 3___ 4___ 5___ >5___ Undetermined___ **NA**___

29. **SUICIDAL ATTEMPTS:**

A. Numbers: 0___ 1___ 2___ 3___ 4___ 5___ >5___ **NA**___

B. Most recent attempt: 1 mo___ <6 mo___ <1 yr___ <5 yr___ >5 yr___ **NA**___

30. **PRESENT ILLNESS:** (Items 31-36) **Reliable**___ Unreliable___

31. **FIRST MANIFESTATION:** <1 yr___ 1-<5 yr___ 5-<10 yr___ >10 yr___ **NA**___

32. **NUMBER OF PREVIOUS EPISODES:**

0___ 1___ 2___ 3___ 4___ 5___ >5___ Undetermined___ NA___

33. COURSE OF ILLNESS:

A. Type: Acute___ Intermittent___ Chronic___ **NA**___

B. Direction: Improving___ Static___ Worsening___ **NA**___

34. PRESENT EPISODE:

A. Duration: >1 wk___ <1 mo___ <6 mo___ <1 yr___ <1 yr___ NA___

B. Symptoms during last week: Lessening___ Static___ Worsening___ NA___

C. Severity during last 3 mo.:

(1) Somatic: Mild___ Moderate___ Severe___ NA___

(2) Psychosocial: Mild___ Moderate___ Severe___ NA___

35. PRIOR TREATMENT (Present episode):

A. Status: Outpt___ Partial Hospitalization___ Inpt___ NA___

B. Psychopharmacological Rx: Neuroleptic___ Antidepressant___ Lithium___ Anxiolytic___ Hypnotic___ Anticonvulsant___ NA___

Other (specify):______________________________

C. Pharmacological Rx: Digitalis___ Antihypertensive___ Antidiabetic___ Geriatric___ NA___

Other (specify):______________________________

D. Nonpharmacological Rx: Psychotherapy___ Social Service___ ECT___ Other____________________ NA___

36. TREATMENT PROVIDER (prior to present admission):

None___ GP___ Internist___ Psychiatrist___ NA___

Other (specify)______________________________

AGP Part 3. Psychopathological Symptoms

CLINIC/HOSP_____ STUDY_____ RATER_____

PT INITIALS_____ PT NO._____ PERIOD____

DATE EXAM___/___/___ STATUS IN__OUT__PART__OTH__
M D Y

SEX M__ F__ RACE W__ B__ I__ O__ OTH__________

BIRTHDATE___/___/___

TIME SPAN RATED TODAY__ <1 wk__ <1 mo__ >1 mo__

AB MI MO SV NA

DIS. CONSCIOUSNES __0

1. Lowered
   0 1 2 3 9
2. Narrowed
   0 1 2 3 9
3. Clouded
   0 1 2 3 9
4. Hypnagogic
   0 1 2 3 9
5. Parasomnia
   0 1 2 3 9

DIS. ORIENTATION __0

6. Time
   0 1 2 3 9
7. Place
   0 1 2 3 9
8. Situation
   0 1 2 3 9
9. Self
   0 1 2 3 9

DIS. ATTENT/MEM. __0

10. Apperception
    0 1 2 3 9
11. Concentration
    0 1 2 3 9
12. Memorization
    0 1 2 3 9
13. Mem. numbers
    0 1 2 3 9
14. Mem. words
    0 1 2 3 9
15. Mem. objects
    0 1 2 3 9

AB MI MO SV NA

16. Mem. forms
    0 1 2 3 9
17. Mem. people
    0 1 2 3 9
18. Mem. colors
    0 1 2 3 9
19. Recent memory
    0 1 2 3 9
20. Remote memory
    0 1 2 3 9
21. Forgetfulness
    0 1 2 3 9
22. Ecmnesia
    0 1 2 3 9
23. Hypermnesia
    0 1 2 3 9
24. Confabulation
    0 1 2 3 9
25. Paramnesias
    0 1 2 3 9
26. Suggestibility
    0 1 2 3 9

DIS. THINKING __0

27. Inhibited
    0 1 2 3 9
28. Retarded
    0 1 2 3 9
29. Circumstantial
    0 1 2 3 9
30. Restricted
    0 1 2 3 9
31. Perseverative
    0 1 2 3 9

AGP Part 3. Psychopathological Symptoms *(continued)*

AB MI MO SV NA

32. Rumination
0 1 2 3 9
33. Pressured
0 1 2 3 9
34. Flight of ideas
0 1 2 3 9
35. Tangential
0 1 2 3 9
36. Blocking
0 1 2 3 9
37. Incoherence
0 1 2 3 9
38. Neologisms
0 1 2 3 9
39. Accelerated
0 1 2 3 9
40. Impaired abstraction
0 1 2 3 9
41. Conceptual impairment
0 1 2 3 9
42. Impaired judgment
0 1 2 3 9

FEARS, COMPULSIONS __0__

43. Suspiciousness
0 1 2 3 9
44. Hypochondriasis
0 1 2 3 9
45. Phobias
0 1 2 3 9
46. Obsess. thoughts
0 1 2 3 9
47. Compul. impulses
0 1 2 3 9
48. Compul. actions
0 1 2 3 9

DELUSIONS __0__

49. Delusional mood
0 1 2 3 9
50. Del. perceptions
0 1 2 3 9
51. Sud. del. thoughts
0 1 2 3 9
52. Delusional idea
0 1 2 3 9
53. System. del
0 1 2 3 9

AB MI MO SV NA

54. Del. dynamics
0 1 2 3 9
55. Del. reference
0 1 2 3 9
56. Del. persecution
0 1 2 3 9
57. Del. jealousy
0 1 2 3 9
58. Del. guilt
0 1 2 3 9
59. Del. impoverish
0 1 2 3 9
60. Hypochond. del.
0 1 2 3 9
61. Del. grandeur
0 1 2 3 9
62. Other del
0 1 2 3 9

DIS. PERCEPTION __0__

63. Illusions
0 1 2 3 9
64. Verbal halluc.
0 1 2 3 9
65. Other auditory
0 1 2 3 9
66. Visual halluc.
0 1 2 3 9
67. Bodily halluc.
0 1 2 3 9
68. Olfact/gust. halluc.
0 1 2 3 9

DIS. EGO __0__

69. Derealization
0 1 2 3 9
70. Depersonalization
0 1 2 3 9
71. Broadcasting
0 1 2 3 9
72. Withdrawal
0 1 2 3 9
73. Insertion
0 1 2 3 9
74. Other influences
0 1 2 3 9

AGP Part 3. Psychopathological Symptoms *(continued)*

AB MI MO SV NA

DIS. AFFECT __0__

75. Perplexity
0 1 2 3 9

76. Loss feeling
0 1 2 3 9

77. Blunted
0 1 2 3 9

78. Loss vitality
0 1 2 3 9

79. Depression
0 1 2 3 9

80. Hopelessness
0 1 2 3 9

81. Anxiety
0 1 2 3 9

82. Euphoria
0 1 2 3 9

83. Dysphoria
0 1 2 3 9

84. Irritability
0 1 2 3 9

85. Inner restless.
0 1 2 3 9

86. Complaintative
0 1 2 3 9

87. Inadequacy
0 1 2 3 9

88. Exag. self-esteem
0 1 2 3 9

89. Feelings of guilt
0 1 2 3 9

90. Impoverishment
0 1 2 3 9

91. Ambivalence
0 1 2 3 9

AB MI MO SV NA

92. Parathymia
0 1 2 3 9

93. Lability
0 1 2 3 9

94. Incontinence
0 1 2 3 9

95. Rigidity
0 1 2 3 9

DIS. DRIVE/MOTILITY __0__

96. Lack drive
0 1 2 3 9

97. Inhibit. drive
0 1 2 3 9

98. Stuporous
0 1 2 3 9

99. Inc. drive
0 1 2 3 9

100. Motor restless.
0 1 2 3 9

101. Parakinesia
0 1 2 3 9

102. Mannerisms
0 1 2 3 9

103. Histrionics
0 1 2 3 9

104. Mutism
0 1 2 3 9

105. Logorrhea
0 1 2 3 9

106. Negativism
0 1 2 3 9

107. Indecisiveness
0 1 2 3 9

AGP Part 4. Psychopathological Symptoms

CLINIC/HOSP_____ STUDY_____ RATER_____

PT INITIALS_____ PT NO._____ PERIOD_____

DATE EXAM____/____/____ STATUS IN__OUT__PART__OTH__
M D Y

SEX M__ F__RACE W__ B__ I__ O__ OTH______________

BIRTHDATE____/____/____
M D Y

TIME SPAN RATED TODAY___ <1 wk___ <1 mo___ >1 mo___

108. PSYCHOORGANIC SYNDROME __0
Site Local___ Diffuse___ NA___
Severity MI___ MO___ SV___ NA___
Duration (yr) <1___ 1<2___ 3<4___ 4<5___ 5<6___
<10___ NA___

AB MI MO SV NA

GLOBAL PERFORMANCE DIS. __0

109. Aphasia
0 1 2 3 9

110. Agnosia
0 1 2 3 9

111. Apraxia
0 1 2 3 9

AB MI MO SV NA

LOCALIZED BRAIN DYSFUNCTION__0

FRONTOPARIETAL DIS. __0

112. Frontal aprax.
0 1 2 3 9

113. Facial aprax.
0 1 2 3 9

114. Prefront. I.S.
0 1 2 3 9

115. Frontobasal I.S.
0 1 2 3 9

116. Motor aphasia
0 1 2 3 9

OCCIPITAL DIS. __0

117. Color/recogn.
0 1 2 3 9

118. Color/naming
0 1 2 3 9

AB MI MO SV NA

119. Color/visual.
0 1 2 3 9

120. Visual agnosia
0 1 2 3 9

121. Prosopagnosia
0 1 2 3 9

122. Dysmorphopsia
0 1 2 3 9

PARIETO-OCCIPITAL DIS. __0

123. Stereoagnosia
0 1 2 3 9

124. Somatagnosia
0 1 2 3 9

125. Anosognosia
0 1 2 3 9

126. Conduction aphasia
0 1 2 3 9

127. Alexia
0 1 2 3 9

128. Agraphia
0 1 2 3 9

129. Acalculia
0 1 2 3 9

130. Ideomotor apraxia
0 1 2 3 9

131. Ideational apraxia
0 1 2 3 9

AGP Part 4. Psychopathological Symptoms *(continued)*

AB MI MO SV NA

132. Construc. apraxia
0 1 2 3 9

TEMPORAL DIS. 0

133. Amnestic aphasia
0 1 2 3 9
134. Sensory aphasia
0 1 2 3 9

CIRCADIAN DIS. 0

135. Worse in AM
0 1 2 3 9
136. Worse in PM
0 1 2 3 9
137. Better in PM
0 1 2 3 9
138. Nighttime exacerb.
0 1 2 3 9
139. Symp. alternation
0 1 2 3 9

DIS. SLEEP/VIGILANCE 0

140. Diff. fall asleep
0 1 2 3 9
141. Interrupt. sleep
0 1 2 3 9
142. Early waking
0 1 2 3 9
143. Prolonged sleep
0 1 2 3 9
144. Shortened sleep
0 1 2 3 9
145. Night restless.
0 1 2 3 9
146. Night confusion
0 1 2 3 9
147. Drowsiness
0 1 2 3 9
148. Day-night reversal
0 1 2 3 9
149. Inc. dreaming
0 1 2 3 9

DIS. SOCIAL BEHAVIOR 0

150. Soc. withdrawal
0 1 2 3 9

AB MI MO SV NA

151. Exces. soc. contact
0 1 2 3 9
152. Aggressiveness
0 1 2 3 9
153. Suicidal
0 1 2 3 9
154. Self-mutilation
0 1 2 3 9
155. Lack feel. ill
0 1 2 3 9
156. Lack insight
0 1 2 3 9
157. Uncooperativeness
0 1 2 3 9
158. Dissimulation
0 1 2 3 9
159. Self-neglect
0 1 2 3 9
160. Refuse nourish.
0 1 2 3 9
161. Dec. libido
0 1 2 3 9
162. Inc. libido
0 1 2 3 9

SOCIAL - NURSING 0

163. Financial needs
0 1 2 3 9
164. Housekeeping
0 1 2 3 9
165. Cont. med. care
0 1 2 3 9
166. Walking
0 1 2 3 9
167. Dressing self
0 1 2 3 9
168. Pers. hygiene
0 1 2 3 9
169. Eating
0 1 2 3 9
170. Leisure activities
0 1 2 3 9
171. Transportation
0 1 2 3 9

AGP Part 4. Psychopathological Symptoms *(continued)*

		AB	MI	MO	SV	NA
172.	Chewing disturb.	0	1	2	3	9
173.	Bedridden	0	1	2	3	9
174.	Urinary incontin.	0	1	2	3	9
175.	Fecal incontin.	0	1	2	3	9
176.	Smearing	0	1	2	3	9

RELIABILITY

0 1 2 3 9

ADDITIONAL EXAMINATIONS _0_

EKG	Y
EEG	Y
Echoencephal-ography	Y
CAT	Y
Scintiscan	Y
Dopplersono-graphy	Y
Angiography	Y
ENG	Y
LP	Y
PEG	Y
EMG	Y
Psych. Tests	Y
RCBF	Y
Other (Specify)	

____

____

AGP Part 5. Somatic Signs

CLINIC/HOSP______ STUDY_____ RATER_____

PT INITIALS______ PT NO._____ PERIOD____

DATE EXAM___/___/___ STATUS IN__OUT__PART__OTH__
M D Y

SEX M__ F__ RACE W__B__I__O__OTH_______________

BIRTHDATE_____/_____/_____
M D Y

---

1. GLOBAL STATE OF HEALTH
   Good_____ Fair_____ Poor_____

AB MI MO SV NA

SOMATIC DISORDERS 0

CARDIOVASCULAR DIS. 0

2. Insufficiency
   0 1 2 3 9
3. Dysrhythmia
   0 1 2 3 9
4. Hypertension
   0 1 2 3 9
5. Other _______________
   0 1 2 3 9
6. RESPIRATORY DIS.
   0 1 2 3 9

GASTROINTESTINAL DIS. 0

7. Hypersalivation
   0 1 2 3 9
8. Dry Mouth
   0 1 2 3 9
9. Nausea
   0 1 2 3 9
10. Constipation
    0 1 2 3 9
11. Diarrhea
    0 1 2 3 9
12. Other _______________
    0 1 2 3 9

UROGENITAL DIS. 0

13. Renal Insuff.
    0 1 2 3 9
14. Micturition dist.
    0 1 2 3 9
15. Other _______________

AB MI MO SV NA

SKELETOMUSCULAR DIS.

16. 0 1 2 3 9

METABOLIC DIS. 0

17. Diabetes mellitus
    0 1 2 3 9
18. Other ____________
    0 1 2 3 9
19. CHRONIC PAIN
    0 1 2 3 9
20. CHRONIC CONSUMPT. PROC.
    0 1 2 3 9

OTHER SOMATIC DIS. 0

21. Blurred vision
    0 1 2 3 9
22. Excessive sweating
    0 1 2 3 9
23. Chills
    0 1 2 3 9
24. Excessive thirst
    0 1 2 3 9
25. Reduced thirst
    0 1 2 3 9
26. Excessive appetite
    0 1 2 3 9
27. Decreased appetite
    0 1 2 3 9
28. Headache
    0 1 2 3 9
29. Dizziness
    0 1 2 3 9
30. Other _______________
    0 1 2 3 9

AGP Part 5. Somatic Signs *(continued)*

NEUROLOGICAL DISORDERS _0_

AB LT BO RT NA

31. OLFACTORY DIS.
0 1 2 3 9

VISION DIS. _0_

32. Central visual
0 1 2 3 9
33. Peripheral visual
0 1 2 3 9
34. Central gaze paresis
0 1 2 3 9
35. Oculomotor paresis
0 1 2 3 9
36. Optokinetic nystagmus
0 1 2 3 9
37. Spontaneous nystagmus
0 1 2 3 9

HEARING DIS. _0_

38. Middle ear
0 1 2 3 9
39. Inner ear
0 1 2 3 9

CENTRAL MOTOR DIS. _0_

40. Hemiparesis
0 1 2 3 9
41. Paraparesis
0 1 2 3 9
42. Quadriparesis
0 1 2 3 9

CENTRAL SENSORY DIS. _0_

43. Hemihypesthesia
0 1 2 3 9
44. Tranverse
0 1 2 3 9

PERIPHERAL MOTOR DIS. _0_

45. Distal
0 1 2 3 9
46. Proximal
0 1 2 3 9
47. PERIPHERAL SENSORY DIS:
0 1 2 3 9

SPINAL CORD LES _0_

AB LT BO RT NA

48. Cervical
0 1 2 3 9
49. Thoracic
0 1 2 3 9
50. Sacrolumbar
0 1 2 3 9

EXTRAPYRAMIDAL DIS. _0_

51. Rigidity
0 1 2 3 9
52. Gross tremor
0 1 2 3 9
53. Fine tremor
0 1 2 3 9
54. Akinesia
0 1 2 3 9
55. Akathisia
0 1 2 3 9
56. Acute dyskinesia
0 1 2 3 9
57. Tardive dyskinesia
0 1 2 3 9

COORDINATION DIS. _0_

58. Intention tremor
0 1 2 3 9
59. Pointing ataxia
0 1 2 3 9
60. Postural ataxia
0 1 2 3 9
61. Gait ataxia
0 1 2 3 9

PRIMITIVE REFLEX _0_

62. Perioral reflex
0 1 2 3 9
63. Grasp reflex
0 1 2 3 9
64. Palmomental reflex
0 1 2 3 9
65. Other ________________
0 1 2 3 9
66. EQUILIBRIUM DIS.
0 1 2 3 9

AGP Part 5. Somatic Signs *(continued)*

AB LT BO RT NA

BULBAR DIS. 0

67. Speaking
0 1 2 3 9

68. Swallowing
0 1 2 3 9

CEREBRAL SEIZURES 0

69. Gen. primary
0 1 2 3 9

70. Gen. secondary
0 1 2 3 9

71. Focal
0 1 2 3 9

72. Unclassified
0 1 2 3 9

AB LT BO RT NA

OTHER CNS 0

73. Peripheral
0 1 2 3 9

74. Central
0 1 2 3 9

75. Psychogenic
0 1 2 3 9

76. HANDEDNESS
0-4 5-9 10-14 9

AGP Part 6. Diagnoses

CLINIC/HOSP_____ STUDY_____ RATER__________

PT INITIALS_____ PT NO.____ PERIOD______

DATE EXAM___/___/___ STATUS IN__OUT__PT__OTH__
M D Y

SEX M__F__ RACE W__B__I__O__Oth__________

BIRTHDATE______/______/______
M D Y

CLINICAL EXPERIENCE (years)

<1__ 1-<3__ 3-<5__ >5__

PSYCHIATRIC DIAGNOSES

ICD-9___ DSM-III___

1. Name______________________

Code______________________

ICD-9 Section: E__ N__ Y__

Diagnostic Certitude: MI__ MO__ HI__

Age at First Manifestation:

0-20__ 21-30__ 31-40__ 41-50__

51-60__ 61-70__ 71-80__ >80__

Certitude (Age): MI__ MO__ HI__

SOMATIC DIAGNOSES None___

1. Name______________________

Code______________________

ICD-9 Section: E___ N___ Y___

Diagnostic Certitude: MI__ MO__ HI__

Age at First Manifestation:

0-20__ 21-30__ 31-40__ 41-50__

51-60__ 61-70__ 71-80__ >80

Certitude (Age): MI__ MO__ HI__

2. Name______________________

Code______________________

ICD-9 Section: E__ N__ Y__

Diagnostic Certitude: MI__ MO__ HI__

Age at First Manifestation

0-20__ 31-30__ 41-50__ 51-60__

51-60__ 61-70__ 71-80__ >80__

Certitude (Age): MI__ MO__ HI__

AGP Part 6. Diagnosis *(continued)*

2. Name______________________________

   Code______________________________

   ICD-9 Section: E__ N__ Y__

   Diagnostic Certitude: MI__ MO__ HI__

   Age at First Manifestation:

   0-20__ 21-30__ 31-40__ 41-50__

   51-60__ 61-70__ 71-80__ >80__

   Certitude (Age): MI__ MO__ HI__

3. Name______________________________

   Code______________________________

   ICD-9 Section: E__ N__ Y__

   Diagnostic Certitude: MI__ MO__ HI__

   Age at First Manifestation

   0-20__ 21-30__ 31-40__ 41-50__

   51-60__ 61-70__ 71-80__ >80__

   Certitude (Age): MI__ MO__HI__

---

3. Name______________________________

   Code______________________________

   ICD-9 Section: E__ N__ Y__

   Diagnostic Certitude: MI__ MO__ HI__

   Age at First Manifestation:

   0-20__ 21-30__ 31-40__ 41-50__

   51-60__ 61-70__ 71-80__ >80__

   Certitude (Age): MI__ MO__ HI__

4. Name______________________________

   Code______________________________

   ICD-9 Section: E__ N__ Y__

   Diagnostic Certitude: MI__ MO__ HI__

   Age at First Manifestation

   0-20__ 21-30__ 31-40__ 41-50__

   51-60__ 61-70__ 71-80__ >80__

   Certitude (Age): MI__ MO__ HI__

Instructions for Raters

Most of the material in this section is based on the special instructions developed for the AMDP system. Given the significant amount of identical content, it seems reasonable and appropriate to utilize the same general "rating set" advocated in that system.

Initial Training

Training procedures specifically designed for the assessment and documentation of the AGP have not yet been developed to the extent of the more established AMDP system. Given the high degree of comparability between the two systems, it is clear that thorough training in the AMDP system can be a valuable – even necessary – introduction to the AGP system. It is strongly recommended, in any case, that neophytes receive instruction and supervision from an experienced AMDP/AGP rater before attempting independent work.

It is important to have the AGP forms at hand while interviewing since they are already "semistructured," i.e., they provide cues for the examiner. While a careful and thorough psychiatric evaluation requires a certain expenditure of time, the completion of Parts 3, 4, and 5 can be substantially accelerated by familiarity with the glossary.

New assessors should be familiar with the AGP definitions of psychopathological and somatic symptoms. This admonition applies not only to the beginner, but to the experienced rater as well. When the latter drifts away from the defined contexts and leans unreflectively upon his own psychopathological conceptualizations, the reliability of his assessments will necessarily be reduced.

Film or videotape presentations of psychiatric interviews to groups of assessors with each assessor completing the AGP forms independently can supplement actual interview experiences. When combined with a discussion of rating inconsistencies, greater motivation among participants and measurable increases in interrater reliability can be attained [5, 7, 18].

At the time of writing, videotapes in English are not yet available. Efforts, however, are underway to assemble a catalogue of interviews which can serve the training needs of English-speaking users of the systems.

Rudiments of Assessment

In assessing psychopathological symptoms the rater makes use of two sources of information: (a) objective data based on direct behavioral observations of his own, of other professional personnel, and of the patient's relatives and (b) subjective data obtained directly from the patient. Diagnostic considerations should not be allowed to prejudice the assessment of specific symptoms. When the assessment is made as part of a multicenter or prospective study, it is recommended that agreement concerning the permissible data sources be reached prior to the initiation of the study.

Every psychopathological assessment evaluates a cross-section of symptoms and behavior present during a specific time span, the duration of which must be held constant throughout any specific investigation. The time span most frequently used is "now or within the last 3 or 4 days" or, in the case of serial examinations, "since the last evaluation." Special circumstances may dictate the use of time spans of different durations. In such cases, however, the time span should be specified to insure that proper interpretation of the data is fostered.

Along with a consistent time span, it is desirable that the rater establish a reasonably uniform framework with which to conduct evaluations. While it is not necessary to adhere to an inflexible assessment routine, the rater should nevertheless endeavor to develop an "interviewing style" which is personally comfortable and productive with most patients. In all cases, however, the rater must be ready to vary his technique to suit unusual circumstances and to maximize the amount of data collected.

The Decision-Making Process

There are four steps in the decision-making process (Fig. 1). The four-step model does not always correspond, however, to the rater's actual psychological process, where the steps may be combined and/or by passed.

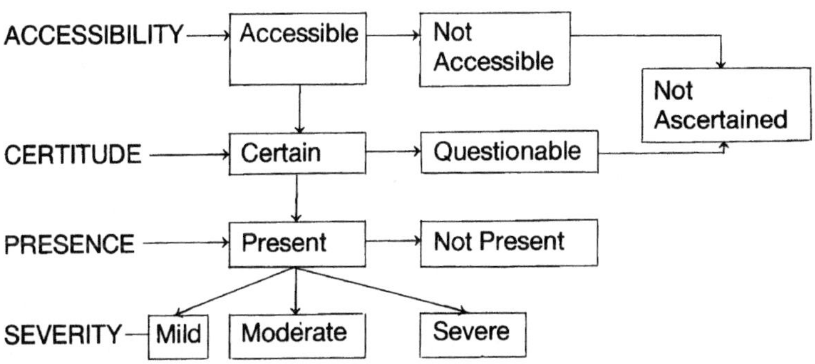

Fig. 1. Decision Tree

1. Accessibility: An item is accessible and thus rateable when the necessary information is available for judgment. A symptom is not accessible (unrateable) when the patient or other informant, despite urging, does not or cannot provide the information necessary for evaluation. In such cases, the item should be encoded as "NA" (not ascertained).

Example: A stuporous or mute patient cannot provide the necessary information for assessing disturbances of orientation, attention, memory, thinking, etc.

2. Certitude: Certitude refers to the confidence the assessor has in the information provided, i.e., in the reliability or certainty of the information. If the assessor is uncertain about the presence or absence of a symptom, i.e., its presence is questionable. "NA" should be encoded.

Example: Negativistic behavior on the part of a patient may cause uncertainty as to whether he is or is not hallucinating.

The response "NA" should not be used to reflect the examiner's personal doubt, but rather the degree of certainty regarding the quality of the information concerning the particular symptom. Both inaccessibility and/or uncertainty may be encoded "NA"; but only after the assessor has made a definite inquiry into every item.

3. Presence: Once the question of certainty has been resolved, the decision concerning the presence or absence of a symptom is made. If the presence of a symptom is questionable, i.e., there is reasonable doubt as to its presence, "NA" should be encoded.

Example: By interviewing a patient suffering from senile dementia, an assessor can usually ascertain the presence or absence of disorientation.

4. Severity: Once a symptom is judged "present," the degree of severity is then estimated as "mild," "moderate," or "severe." This judgment is based on a combination of intensity, significance, and frequency.

Examples of these encoding procedures are given in Table 1. Careful and complete encoding of every item is very important for subsequent analyses.

After the completion of the interview, the examiner should recheck the assessment forms for errors, ambiguities, or omissions. When correcting an entry, it should be ensured that the correction can be distinguished from the error, i.e., by thorough erasure or by a clear deletion mark.

Table 1. Encoding Procedures

	AD	MI	MO	SV	NA
a) Dis. Consciousness ⓪					
b) Lowered	⓪	1	2	3	9
c) Narrowed	0	1	2	3	⑨
d) Clouded	0	1	②	3	9
e) Hynagogic	0	1	2	3	⑨
Parasomnia	0	1	2	3	9

Examples	*Response*
a) None of the 5 symptoms under *"Disorders of Consciousness"* are present	Circle "0" (absent) beside the major heading.
b) The symptom *"Lowered Consciousness"* is absent.	Circle "0" (absent) for the item.
c) The symptom *"Narrowed Consciousness"* cannot be assessed.	Circle "9" (NA) for the item.
d) The symptom *"Clouded Consciousness"* is present to a moderate degree.	Circle "2" (moderate) for the item.
e) The symptom *"Hypnagogic States"* is questionably present.	Circle "9" (NA) for the item.

The Scaling of Psychopathological Symptoms

Greater agreement among raters on the presence or absence of a symptom is more likely when regular and continuous practice in evaluation and documentation occurs (7, 18). Symptoms which show a gradual transition from health to disturbance are much more difficult to judge "present" or "absent" than those which show a sudden and dramatic emergence.

Substantially more difficult than the judgment of presence/absence is the grading of a symptom along the severity continuum "mild," "moderate," and "severe." Since both intensity and duration of a symptom enter into the judgment, it follows that, under the condition of marked prominence but short duration, a symptom may be mistakenly rated "mild". Symptoms of lesser prominence but more constantly present may be rated too high. In other words, "mild but continually present" can receive the same rating as "severe but transiently present". In such cases, the intensity of the experience and/or behavior should be given precedence, especially since the usual observational timeframe is so brief, i.e., a few days. With fluctuating symptoms, the highest intensity within the timeframe should be rated.

With longer observation periods (several weeks), the combining of intensity, duration, and frequency into a single judgment is more difficult and and optimal solution has not yet been found. For standardization, however, it is recommended that less prominent, constantly present symptoms be rated "mild," and occasionally present (perhaps only once) symptoms of great intensity, "moderate" – so as to leave the judgment of "severe" for the frequently present symptom of great intensity.

The definitions provided in the glossary first describe the nature and dimensions of the symptom and then give examples which illustrate the two anchor points of "mild" and "severe." This was not always possible for every symptom and, therefore, some definitions may seem forced or arbitrary.

On "Deviation from the Norm"

For most symptoms, the boundary of health is often unclear and not easily defined. As a result, subjective interpretation by the rater is unavoidable. To judge deviation from health, it is necessary to decide which of several norms should be used: a general cultural norm, a special norm for the sociocultural stratum of the patient (or the investigator!), or the individual norm of the patient? Even if the intraindividual difference between the patient's premorbid and morbid state is known, the investigator should give it no weight in the judgment of the severity of the AGP symptom. Rather, the transition from health to pathology experienced by the patient and/or observed by the rater should be assessed according to its deviation from the general (societal) norm. Comparisons involving the time factor should be avoided. Thus, the assessment of a symptom in the AGP system does not differentiate a personality or disposition variable (trait) from a disease or condition variable (state).

The Synthesis of Subjective Experience and Objective Findings

A combination of "subjective" and "objective" information is utilized for all AGP evaluations. This confluence of information from the patient's description of his disturbance and from external observation can create problems. This is especially true in judgments of immediate memory, retention, concentration, etc. For example, a depressive patient without apparent memory disturbance but, in consequence of his retardation, with feelings of inadequacy and low self-esteem, complains about the slackening of his memory power or, in his depressed mood, calls himself stupid although actually of average intelligence. In such a case, judgment is to be based on the objective findings since the AGP symptom glossary is not meant to be a complaint list. At the same time, however, Item 87 – "Feelings of Inadequacy" – would be rated. When, however, the patient's subjective complaints cannot be substantiated objectively, e.g., complaints, at admission, of disturbed sleep and constipation, the symptom must be rated chiefly on the patient's subjective report. In some cases the synthesis of subjective and objective data components can be resolved by rating two symptoms, one reflecting the subjective experience and the other the observed behavior; e.g., Item 27 – "Inhibited Thinking" – vs Item 28 – "Retarded Thinking" –, where the assessment of inhibition is based on subjective experience and retardation on observations by the rater.

The Identification Block

To identify data collected from an individual patient at a single examination and to prevent loss of such data, each of the separate AGP assessment sheets has the same basic information block (ID) printed at the top of the sheet. Complete and accurate encoding of the ID block is necessary for the collection of material and the subsequent data processing and analyses. Since experience has shown that errors of omission and commission within the ID block are a major problem in data editing, raters are urged to be particularly conscientious in completing this block.

The items comprising the ID block are:

1. Part Number: A number for each of the six AGP sections is preprinted, along with the title, at the top of the page.

2. Clinic/Hosp: The name (or number) of the clinic, hospital, or other facility conducting the study.

3. Study: The name (or number) of the study, trial, or investigation in which the patient is a participant.

4. Rater: The name (or number of the rater (assessor) conducting the examination and/or completing the particular section.

5. Status: The designation of the patient's status at the time of the examination. Inpatient (In) refers to 24-hour hospitalization. Outpatient (Out) refers to nondomiciliary treatment. Partial hospitalization (Part) refers to treatment programs involving a significant portion of a 24-hour period, e.g., day hospital, night hospital.

6. Patient Initials: Two initials – given (first) name followed by surname (last) name – are encoded to aid in data collection. To maintain confidentiality, the patient's full name should not be entered.

7. Patient Number: A number assigned to a given patient throughout a given study and employed later in data processing as an anonymous designator. This number must be uniformly encoded on all AMDP parts for all evaluations.

8. Period: In a series of evaluations on a given patient, a number designating the sequential position of a particular examination; i.e., 1st, 2nd, 3rd, etc. For most studies with repeated ratings, evaluations are designated by the day of the study; i.e., day 00 (the initial or pretreatment day), 07, 14, etc. A single assessment of a patient is also designated as "00." The encoding of "Period" must be uniform for all ratings within a single study.

9. Date of Examination: The date (month-day-year) on which the examination occurred. Since information for Parts 1, 2, and 3 often may be collected over several days, it is suggested that uniform dating be established for these sessions, i.e., the three anamnestic parts should all be dated alike.

10. Sex: Male (M) or female (F) (initial examination only).

11. Race: One entry at initial examination only. The races are: white (W), black (B), amerind (I), oriental (O), and other (to be specified). Mixed heritage should be encoded under "other".

12. Birthdate: The patient's birthdate (month-day-year) is encoded at initial examination only. Partial information, e.g., year of birth, should be encoded, if that is all the information available.

When all AGP parts are used as a unit, these data are sufficient for identification. If the sections are used independently, e.g., only Parts 3 and 4, it may be necessary to supplement data by gathering basic demographic information.

Glossary

The Anamnesis (Part 1 and 2)

The AGP Anamnesis consists of two sections:

Part 1 – Demographic Data (two assessment sheets)
Part 2 – Psychiatric History (two assessment sheets)

The two-part Anamnesis requires an expenditure of considerable time and effort. In return, however, an extensive set of sociodemographic data is obtained with which to supplement the psychiatric findings. While it is possible to use the parts independently, it is suggested that both anamnestic parts be completed at the initial examination for every patient. Most items refer to status at the time of the examination or, in the case of inpatients, status prior to present admission.

To facilitate the encoding of the anamnestic sections, the following general codes are employed:

NA = Not ascertained, not assessed, not applicable, not answered. This response position is present for all anamnestic items. It is a general "missing data" code and should be used only after unsuccessful or unsatisfactory inquiry has been made.
Y = Yes
N = No

The number of permissible entries is given for each item, e.g., "One entry only" or "Multiple entries permitted," and must not be exceeded by the examiner. To do so will hamper subsequent data processing by increasing the number of errors of commission.

Most anamnestic items are completed by making a check (✓,x) on the line following the appropriate response.

Example: 23. Type of Admission: Voluntary ✓ Involuntary ___
NA ___

Other items require a numerical entry.

Example: 2. Age: 75 NA ___

When making corrections, cross out the incorrect response and circle the correct one.

Example: 11. Residential Setting: Urban ✓ Suburban ~~✓~~
Rural ___ NA ___

Part 1 – Demographic Data

The Demographic data consist of 24 items dealing primarily with personal historical information, e.g., age, marital status, and employment. A variety of sources may be used to obtain the necessary data, including the patient, family members, friends, and medical and social agencies. Part 1 may be completed by paraprofessionals, but responsibility for the accuracy of the data rests with the psychiatric assessor.

1. Source of Anamnesis: One entry only. "Primary" indicates that almost all the data were freshly gathered, i.e., directly at the time of the examination. "Secondary" indicates that almost all the data were gathered from extramural sources, i.e., indirectly from previous records or documentations. "Both" indicates that substantial parts of the information were obtained from both primary and secondary sources.

2. Age: A two-digit numerical entry. Encode age in years at the time of the interview.

3. Marital Status: One entry only. Refers to status at the time of the examination. The choices are:

Single = never married
Mar'd = married, legal
Sep'd = separated, living apart by choice or legal decree
Div. = divorced

Widw = widowed
Cohab = cohabiting, legally unmarried. "Single" (1) and "Cohabiting" (6) are not mutually exclusive. When both are applicable, encode "Cohabiting" (6).
NA = not ascertained

4. *Nationality:* One entry only. Refers to the patient's citizenship status in relation to the country in which the examination is conducted. The choices are:
Citizen by birth
Naturalized: granted citizenship by legal process
Alien: noncitizen of host country
Stateless: without legal citizenship status in any country
NA: not ascertained

Examples: A patient born in Boston and residing in Nashville at the time of the examination should be encoded "Citizen by birth." A Canadian citizen residing in Nashville at the time of the interview should be encoded "Alien."

5. *Children:* A two-part item.
A. Number: One entry for the total number of the patient's children. Include both biological and adoptive/foster children.
B. Presently Living: One entry for the number of the patient's children alive at the time of the examination.

6. *Siblings:* A three-part item.
A. Number: One entry for the total number of siblings. Both adoptive and foster siblings are included along with biological siblings.
B. Presently Living: One entry for the number of siblings alive at the time of the interview.
C. Twins: One entry for multiple births, e.g., twins, triplets.

7. *Religion:* One entry only. Refers to membership or adherence at the time of the examination. This item may be deleted

at the discretion of the investigator if it is considered an invasion of privacy. The choices are:

Protestant
Roman Catholic
Hebrew
None: includes atheists, agnostics, and unaffiliated believers
Other: specify sect

8. Religious Conviction: One entry only. An estimate of the intensity of the patient's religious or philosophical ties to the sect entered in Item 7. Rate as "weak," "average," or "strong".

9. Trusteeship: One entry only. Refers to the establishment of a trust for the patient's affairs.

10. Guardianship: One entry only. Refers to the appointment of a legal guardian for the patient's affairs.

11. Residential Setting: One entry only. The choices are:
Urban: central metropolitan areas, large cities
Suburban: communities adjacent to metropolitan areas
Rural: small towns, villages, farms

12. Residential Status:
A. Present Residence: One entry only. Refers to the residence of the patient at the time of the examination. For inpatient settings, patient's residence prior to admission should be encoded. The choices are:

- *Own Home*: Includes home, apartment, or condominium owned by patient or his family.
- *Rental Accommodation:* Includes rental home or duplex as well as apartment.
- *Subtenancy:* Includes subleases of room or part of an apartment.
- *Independent Geriatric Setting:* Dwelling specially designed or designated for the elderly in which provision for

independent housekeeping is made. Some provision for health care may be available.

– *Supervised Geriatric Setting:* Establishments for the elderly not in need of total nursing care but who are not able to maintain their own independent household without external assistance and supervision.

– *Nursing Home:* Institutions for the care of persons, including chronically ill geriatric patients, who require continuous supervision and/or medical care.

– *General/Psychiatric Hospital:* Includes all medical, psychiatric or special hospitals in which constant medical service is provided for physical and/or psychiatric illness.

– *No Fixed Address:* Refers to persons without an established residence, e.g., those living on the street or in "flophouses," squatters.

– *Other:* Includes any type of residence not encompassed by the above.

B. Institutional Residence: One or two entries permitted. Refers to institutional residence at the time of the examination, e.g., independent or supervised geriatric setting, nursing home, hospital. If only the patient is residing in an institution, encode "pat." If only the patient's spouse is institutionalized, encode "spouse." If patient and spouse are both residing in the same institution, encode "pt/spouse." If patient and spouse are "institutionalized" in different institutions, encode "pat" and "spouse" separately.

13. Household Composition (excluding patient): Multiple entries permitted. Include all persons who are living together and sharing the household at the time of the examination. The choices are:

Spouse: unmarried partner (common law) as well as legally married spouse

Children: adoptive and stepchildren as well as biological ones

Siblings: adoptive and stepsiblings as well as biological ones

Parents: as above
Grandchildren: as above
Others: all other relatives and/or nonrelatives
NA: not ascertained

14. Household Income: A three-part item. Household income, is defined as the total income of the family unit.
A. Level: One entry only. "Dependent" is defined as the major portion of income derived from external (nonfamily) sources, either public or private, e.g., welfare, social, or charitable agencies. "Marginal" is defined as minimal subsistence level derived primarily from internal (family) sources. "Adequate" is defined as an adequate as well as abundant level of income.
B. Source: Multiple entries permitted. The choices are:

Pension: retirement benefits including Social Security, VA, etc.
Salary: income from present full – or part-time work
Capital Assets: income from property, interest, dividends, etc.
Social Agency: income from governmental or private agencies due to incapacitation and/or dependency
Other: any other sources of income
NA: not ascertained

C. Number Supported: One entry only. Total number of persons, including the patient, supported by this income.

15. Education: One entry only. Encode the highest level (complete or partial) attained by the patient. It is presumed that the lower levels were completed. The choices are:
Special Education: special or ungraded education for retarded or handicapped
Elementary: kindergarten through grade 8
High School: grades 9 – 12
College: undergraduate college or university, junior college
Graduate School: including professional schools, e.g., medicine, law, dentistry
NA: not ascertained

16. Vocational Training: One entry may be made for both "Apprenticeship" and "Business/Technical School." "Apprenticeship" refers to supervised job experience leading to qualification as a craftsman, e.g., plumber, carpenter, mason. "Business/Technical School" refers to specialized training in nonacademic institutions, e.g., secretarial, accounting, computer programming.

17. Occupation: A two-part item.
A. Level: Encode the highest level ever reached and the level of the last job held for both the patient and spouse. A maximum of four entries is permitted. If the spouse is deceased, enter occupational level achieved prior to death. For the "never married" patient, encode NA under both "Spouse" columns. The choices are:

Homemaker: Refers to full-time housekeeping – by either male or female – as the major occupational duty actively engaged in prior to reaching retirement, provided more than one person is being cared for

Homemaker – 2nd job: Dual function as housekeeper with gainful employment

Student: Participant in formal educational program

Self-employed Worker: Independent tradesman or worker (not a wage earner or salaried employee) with at least one employee. Includes the independent small farmer

Self-employed Entrepreneur: Independent small businessman. May employ other workers. Small store owner, barber shop owner, appliance repair shop owner, etc.

Major Professional: Directors and executives of large public or private enterprises, physicians, lawyers, university faculty

Minor Professional: Intermediate (middle) level executives or managers, registered nurses, elementary teachers, pharmacists, etc.

Skilled Worker: Craftsman, foreman, supervisor

Semiskilled Worker: Machine operators, clerical workers

Unskilled Worker: Manual laborers, busboy, domestic service

NA: Not ascertained

B. Presently Unemployed: One entry only. Refers to total unemployment; e.g., patient with part-time, gainful work would be encoded "No," i.e., not unemployed.

18. Retirement: A three-part item.
A. The status of the patient at the time of the examination: "Retired usual" refers to retirement at the standard Social Security age of 65. "Retired early" refers to retirement prior to the usual age of 65 for any reason. "Retired late" refers to retirement delayed beyond the usual age. One entry only.
B. The circumstances of the retirement: "Involuntary" refers to any enforced retirement; i.e., against the patient's will. Encode NA if patient is not retired.

19. Freetime Activities: One entry only. Refers to unpaid, spontaneous activities, e.g., participant or spectator sports, hobbies.

20. Social Relationships: A two-part item.
A. Objective: A quantitative estimate by the examiner of the degree (extent) of the patient's social interactions.
B. Subjective: A qualitative estimate by the patient of the degree of satisfaction obtained from social interaction.

21. Previous Care: Multiple entries are permitted. All persons or agencies which provided care to the patient at the time of the examination. The choices are:

None: no previous care and/or treatment
Spouse: legal or common law
Family: any relative except spouse
Friend: nonrelatives, neighbors, etc.
Charitable/Religious Organizations: Private secular or religious agencies
Health Facility: public or private
Other Governmental Agency: public nonmedical agency
Other (specify): any person or agency not encompassed by the above
NA: not ascertained

22. Referral Source: Multiple entries permitted. Include all persons and/or institutions involved in the referral. The choices are:

Self
Spouse/family
Physician
Clinic/hosp
Service agency
Other (specify)
NA: not ascertained

23. Type of Admission: One entry only. "Voluntary" refers to admission by the patient's free choice. "Involuntary" refers to any form of legal commitment.

24. Reason for Commitment: One entry only. Encode the basis for the present commitment. (Voluntary admission is encoded "NA.") The choices are:

Suicidal Attempt: actual life-threatening actions
Dangerous to Self: includes suicide threats, self-mutilation, life-threatening gestures
Dangerous to Others: includes homicidal/assaultive acts or threats, behavior which endangers the safety of others
Other (specify)
NA: not ascertained

Part 2 – Psychiatric History

"Psychiatric History" consists of 12 items dealing primarily with the patient's history, family psychiatric history, past treatment, and present episode. The items of Part 2 are numbered in sequence from Part 1; i.e., from Item 25 to Item 36. To a greater extent than Part 1, Part 2 requires judgments which are best made by the psychiatric examiner rather than paraprofessionals.

25. Family Psychiatric Illness: A two-part item. First degree relative refers to parents, children, siblings, half-siblings. Distant relative refers to 2nd and 3rd degree relatives; e.g., aunts, uncles, cousins. The choices are:

None: no known psychiatric illness
Suspected: a psychiatric illness is probable but clear-cut evidence or diagnosis is not available
Confirmed: a psychiatric illness with supportive evidence, but without hospitalization
Hospitalized: a confirmed psychiatric illness for which hospitalization was required
NA: not ascertained

26. Previous Nonpsychiatric Illness: A multipart item with multiple entries permitted. If the patient has had no previous non psychiatric diseases – "CNS" or "Other Organ" – check both spaces and leave the rest of the item blank:

No CNS _✓_ Other Organ _✓_ diseases

If the patient has had a nonpsychiatric CNS disease but no "Other Organ" disease, encode as follows and complete appropriate CNS subitems.

No CNS ____ Other Organ _✓_ disease

Should the converse be true, encode as follows and complete appropriate "Other Organ" subitems.

No CNS _✓_ Other Organ ____ disease

For any disease which the patient has experienced, a maximum of two entries is permitted, e.g., "suspected" and "sequelae" or "confirmed" and "sequelae." "Suspected" and "confirmed" are defined in Item 25. "Sequelae" refers to any residual effects or persistence of the disease which are present at the time of the examination. The diseases cited are:

CNS	Other Organ
Inflammatory	*Inflammatory*
Trauma	*Trauma*
Constitutional	*Constitutional*
Intoxication: either endogenous or exogenous	*Intoxication:* either endogenous or exogenous

Epilepsy: either primary or traumatic
Surgical

Metabolic: with significant clinical symptoms
Cardiovascular
Surgical

27. Previous Psychiatric Illness: A multipart item in which multiple entries are permitted. Encode as in Item 26. The diseases cited are:

None: indicates that the patient had no history of any of the diseases listed below.
Constitutional/childhood illness: "Inborn" or other psychiatric disorders in childhood
Endogenous psychoses
Exogenous psychoses
Psychoneurotic reactions
Addiction: If addiction is encoded as "suspected," "confirmed" and/or "sequelae," encode the type(s) of addiction:
Addiction:
Alcohol
Hypnotic/analgesic
Opiate
Other
NA: not ascertained

28. Number of Previous Psychiatric Admissions: One entry only. Refers to 24-hour and partial hospitalizations, exclusive of present admission. Do not count outpatient admissions. "Undetermined" is encoded when previous hospitalizations are known to have occurred, but the exact number is unknown. Encode "NA" when information is unobtainable or unreliable.

29. Suicidal Attempts: A two-part item.
A. Number: One entry only. Encode the total number of attempts, including one which may have precipitated the present admission. If there have been no attempts, encode "0" and leave 29B blank.

B. Most recent attempt: One entry only. Indicate the time elapsed since most recent (last) attempt.

30. Present Illness: One entry only. If the following information concerning the present illness or episode (Items 31–36) is considered unreliable, insufficient, or unobtainable, check "Unreliable." Items 31–36 may still be encoded, but they will be considered as specious data.

31. First Manifestation: One entry only. Estimate the time span between first manifestation and the present, i.e., time of examination.

32. Number of Previous Episodes: One entry only. Estimate the number of prior episodes, excluding the present episode. If prior episodes are known to have occurred but the exact number is unknown, encode "undetermined." Encode "NA" when information is unobtainable or unreliable.

33. Course of Illness: A two-part item.
A. Type: One entry only. "Acute" refers to a new or early phase of illness or an acute exacerbation of a chronic condition. "Intermittent" refers to a fluctuating or phasic condition. "Chronic" refers to static, longstanding condition.
B. Direction: One entry only. Refers to overall course of the illness.

34. Present Episode: A three-part item.
A. Duration: One entry only. Estimate the duration of the present episode from its beginning to the time of the examination.
B. Symptoms during last week: One entry only. Estimate the course of the symptomatology for this time span, i.e., lessening, static, or worsening.
C. Severity during last 3 months: One entry only. Estimate the degree of impairment or dysfunction of the patient's somatic (1) and psychosocial (2) condition over the stated time span.

35. Prior Treatment (Present Episode): A four-part item. Refers to treatments preceding examination but related to the present episode only.

A. Status: Multiple entries permitted. Encode all facilities involved. "Outpatient" (Outpt) refers to nondomiciliary care. "Partial Hospitalization" (Part. Hosp.) refers to treatment programs involving a significant portion of a 24-hour period, e.g., day hospital, night hospital. "Inpatient" (Inpt) refers to 24-hour hospitalization.

B. Psychopharmacological Rx: Multiple entries permitted. Encode all classes of psychotropics involved in episode. The choices are:

Neuroleptic
Antidepressant
Lithium
Anxiolytic
Hypnotic/sedative
Anticonvulsant
Other (specify)
NA: not ascertained

C. Pharmacological Rx: Multiple entries permitted. Encode all classes of nonpsychotropic medication involved. The choices are:

Digitalis
Antihypertensive
Antidiabetic
Geriatric
Other (specify)
NA: non ascertained

D. Nonpharmacological Rx: Multiple entries permitted. Encode all nondrug treatments involved. The choices are:

Psychotherapy: individual or group of any "school," behavior modification etc.
Social Service: all types of service and/or assistance
Electroconvulsive Rx (ECT): all forms of ECT
Other (specify)
NA: not ascertained

36. Treatment Provider (prior to present admission): Multiple entries permitted. The choices are:

None: no previous treatment
General Practitioner (GP)
Internist
Psychiatrist
Other (specify)
NA: not ascertained

Psychopathological Symptoms

"Psychopathological Symptoms" consists of 176 items organized in two sections:

Part 3 – nine symptom clusters, 107 symptoms
Part 4 – nine symptom clusters, 69 symptoms

Together, the parts provide the basis for a comprehensive evaluation of psychopathology in the geriatric patient. The congruence of the AGP system with the AMDP-III system can be demonstrated by the fact that 104 AMDP-III symptoms along with their definitions are contained within Parts 3 and 4 of the AGP. Given this common ground, the two systems provide a substantial data base for the study of psychopathology across the life span, i.e., from adult through geriatric years. Symptoms common to both the AMDP-III and the AGP are designated by citing their AMDP-III item number in parentheses following the definition of the symptom.

Each symptom has been carefully defined to provide a uniform context for assessment. It is imperative that raters be thoroughly familiar with the definitions provided and rate each item within its contextual framework.

To encode a judgment of a symptom, the rater circles the appropriate degree of severity.

Ex. AB MI (MO) SV MA

When all symptoms listed under a major heading, i.e., cluster, are absent, the rater need only circle the "zero" beside the heading and proceed to the next heading.

Part 3 – Psychopathological Symptoms

To a great extent, this section corresponds to "AMDP Part III: Psychopathological Symptoms" – 80% of the symptoms appear in both sections. These symptoms, for the most part, are common in both adult and geriatric populations and, simultaneously, cover the major portion of the psychopathological spectrum.

Time Span Rated

This item precedes the catalogue of symptoms. It permits the rater to designate the time period encompassed by the examination. The choices provided are:

Today: A point-in-time evaluation essentially restricted to symptomatology present during the examination or within the past 24 hour.

One week or less: The most frequently used time span. Closely approximates the time span advocated in AMDP-III, i.e., "now or within the last 3 or 4 days."

One month or less

More than 1 month: These latter two spans are more applicable for the initial examination.

For repeated examinations such as those conducted during a clinical psychotropic drug trial, the time span is frequently defined as "since the last examination."

Disorders of Consciousness

In this category, degrees of disturbance in one's total experience and overall behavior are assessed, including disturbances in activity, clarity of one's perceptions and intentions, purposefulness of conduct, attentiveness, apperception, conversational responsiveness, reactivity, adaptiveness in thinking, will, and behavior, and vigilance. Qualitative disturbances of consciousness such as narrowing or distortions and quantitative disturbances such as changes in vigilance are frequently combined in the assessment of severity.

1. Lowered Vigilance: A rise in the threshold of all incoming stimuli; decreased responsiveness to environmental contingencies or reduction of vigilance. Lowered consciousness ranges from decreased mental clarity or "in a daze" *(Benommenheit)* – which scores "mild" – through somnolence ("moderate") to sopor, precoma, and coma ("severe"). The patient is apathetic, slowed down, drowsy, and keeps dosing off; he or she is easily awakened in somnolence but only with great difficulty in sopor. (AMDP-III, 1)

2. Narrowed Consciousness: Constriction of that which enters into awareness. This comes about by fixation on or fascination with certain inner and outer experiences or events. Characteristic of narrowed consciousness is the diminished reactivity to external events, i.e., shutting oneself off from stimuli. (AMDP-III, 3)

3. Clouded Consciousness: Twilight state. Dreamlike confusional states, e.g., predelirium, delirium, oneiroid states. Disturbances of consciousness with varying and fluctuating degrees of severity – often with increasing psychomotor activity, partial or total disorientation, incoherent thinking, and illusionary misinterpretations of the surroundings. Various, fluctuating experiences occur, from dreamlike confusion to fleeting delusions and hallucinations (these are usually optical, but sometimes other sensory systems are involved). Reactivity to stimulation from the environment is usually intact. Disturbances of the sleep/wake system are usually disturbances of the autonomic system.

4. Hypnagogic States: Mild reductions in vigilance, usually upon going to sleep or upon waking; often accompanied by dreamlike imagery or pseudohallucinations.

5. Parasomnia: A special consciousness disturbance like the apallic syndrome. This expression was introduced by Kretschmer about 1930 to denote a condition in which the patient lies motionless with the eyes open, apparently awake but without fixing the gaze on moving objects as in stupor, and does not turn attention to external stimuli. This condition may lead to coma or death; however, remission is possible, but is often accompanied by permanent mental damage. Kretschmer felt the condition is caused by an interruption between cerebrum and brain stem in the pallidum (lentiform nucleus of the brain). This interpretation is more current in European psychiatry than in modern neurology; the latter discipline interprets the condition as a form of frontal akinesia. The examiner cannot ascertain how much of the "psychological life" of the patient is still preserved. Alternations of sleep and waking states are present.

Disturbances of Orientation

Disorientation refers to the inability to recognize or evaluate accurately temporal, spatial, or personal situations as they occur.

6. Time: Lack of awareness of day, month, year, or season. By convention, patients with memory disturbances who cannot order their past history in the correct chronological sequence are not included here. It is not uncommon for patients (or nonpatients for that matter) to be imprecise in stating the numerical date, i.e., to be 1 or 2 days "off" from the actual date. Such deviations should be judged leniently. (AMDP-III, 5).

7. Place: Lack of awareness of one's location. Patient does not know where he is, i.e., inability to identify one's present location. (AMDP-III, 6)

8. Situation: Inability to assess correctly the surroundings and one's place in it, e.g., a patient being examined by the doctor. Delusional disorientation may be entered here, e.g., delusional misinterpretation of situations. (AMDP-III, 7)

9. Self: Lack of awareness of one's identity. Patient does not know his name and/or misconstrues his personal history. (AMPD-III, 8)

Example: An old man knows his name, but feels himself to be a young boy who is just going shopping for his grandmother.

Disturbances of Attention and Memory

Disturbances of apperception, concentration, and memory are assessed under this heading. Attention and memory disturbances are to be rated here only if they are objectifiable manifestations – not just subjective feelings – of impaired apperception, concentration, and memory. If the examiner is unable to find concrete evidence of impairment or obtain a credible report of such deficiencies from the patient, only Item 87, "Feelings of Inadequacy," should be rated.

10. Apperception: The inability to grasp the meaning and significance of experience or to see the meaningful connections between them. In a broader sense the inability to integrate new experiences with one's own past experience. Apperception may be inappropriate, delayed, or absent. One has to evaluate clinically whether the behavior is congruent with the situation. Psychological testing through use of TAT, short stories, proverbs, etc. may be required. If the disturbance is the result of sensory aphasia, rate under "Psychopathological Symptoms – Part 4." (AMDP-III, 9)

11. Concentration: The inability to focus on a topic and remain focused. Failure to keep one's attention on a specific matter or objective for a reasonable time. In everyday language, attention span or the inability "to stick to a task." (AMDP-III, 10)

12. Memorization: Disturbed immediate memory. The partial or total inability to retain *freshly acquired* material for more than 10 min. This may be tested by asking the patient to repeat a series of numbers or sentences, to recognize objects, etc., after a lapse of 10 min. Immediate memory impairment may vary from one sense modality to another and from one subject or object to another and is also dependent upon the emotional state of the patient or the emotional loading of the material presented. Hence, it is better to use neutral material when testing. (AMDP-III, 11)

If only a global assessment of disturbed memory is to be made, a single response to Item 12 will suffice. In this case, Items 13–18 are encoded "NA", i.e., not assessed. If a more detailed testing of memory impairment is undertaken, Items 13–18 should be encoded individually.

13. Memorization for Numbers

14. Memorization for Words

15. Memorization for Objects

16. Memorization for Forms

17. Memorization for People

18. Memorization for Colors

19. Recent Memory: In a broad sense, impaired memory for events of the recent past; i.e., minutes, hours, or days. This item has been operationally differentiated from Item 12, "Memorization," by restricting Item 12 to impairment of narrowly circumscribed tasks, e.g., retention of recently dictated numbers, words, etc., while assessing the present item in the broader context of disturbed memory for the events of daily life. Severity is rated according to the following criteria.

– *Mild (MI):* Small memory lapses for actual daily events in a generally sound memory system.

– *Moderate (MO):* Significant, marked lapses for daily events in a partially impaired memory system.

– *Severe (SV):* Isolated memory traces for daily events in an almost totally dysfunctional memory system.

20. Remote Memory: Impaired memory for events of the distant past, i.e., months, years. Criteria for judging severity are:

Mild (MI): A few pathological lapses for distant past events.

Moderate (MO): Significant, marked gaps for distant past events but with partial memory retention.

Severe (SV): In spite of isolated memory traces, an almost total loss of memory for distant past events.

21. Increased Forgetfulness: Forgetting earlier information when immediately thereafter new material is presented, i.e., interspersed between presentation and recall.

Example: In testing word memory, inability to recall the first word in the list after the second word is given.

22. Ecmnesia: Disturbance of time sense, i.e., incorrect temporal sequence, in which the past experiences are placed or ordered, e.g., the past is experienced as the present. Seen in senile memory loss, clouded consciousness, and certain emotionally loaded states. (This item is subsumed under AMDP-III, 14 – "Paramnesia.")

23. Hypermnesia (Remote Memory): Very lively and precise remembrance, in all detail, of long past experiences. "Telescopage." (Subsumed under AMDP-III, 14.)

24. Confabulation: The filling of memory gaps with reports of imagined or supposedly experienced events which the patient regards as real. The content of confabulation for the same memory gap can change continually. This last point is important for differentiation from pseudologia fantastica. (AMDP-III, 13)

25. Paramnesias: False or altered memories. Also delusional memories in which the remembrance is transformed by delusional thinking. Never-experienced recognitions (déjà-vu) or unrecognized previous experiences (jamais-vu) are rated here. In déjà-vu, the patient reacts as though everything presently seen has been seen and experienced before in exactly the same way, down to the last detail. Conversely, jamais-vu consists of reacting to everything as though it is seen for the first time; everything is unfamiliar, fresh, or incomprehensible. (AMDP-III, 4 encompasses this item as well as AGP-21 and AGP-23.)

26. Suggestibility: Increased susceptibility to external influence of thoughts, feelings, will, and behavior so that these functions are not regulated and controlled to the usual degree by the patient.

Formal Disorders of Thought

27. Inhibited Thinking: Experienced by the patient as slowing-down (braking), unevenness, or faltering in the thinking process as if due to the presence of obstacles. The inhibition in tempo, content, or goal-directedness cannot be removed, however hard the patient tries. Inhibited thinking, in contrast to Item 28, "Retarded Thinking," has to be subjectively experienced. (AMDP-III, 15)

28. Retarded Thinking: Slow, laborious flow of thought processes. Continuous delays in expressing thoughts with almost no progress. The viscosity and torpidity in speech and reactions are observable to the rater. Retardation must be differentiated from Item 27 ("Inhibited Thinking") and Item 31 ("Perseveration"). (AMDP-III, 16)

29. Circumstantial Thinking: Inability to differentiate the essential from the unessential: getting lost in significant details without losing track of the question. Circumstantiality may be the result of loss of abstract ability or the result of an inability to omit insignificant details even when they are recognized as such, e.g., pedantry, pettyfogging. Rate only if the progress of the examination is hindered by the rambling thoughts. Item 37 ("Incoherence") is not rated here. (AMDP-III, 17)

30. Restricted Thinking: Poverty of ideas. Characterized by shrinking of the thought content and fixation on a few themes only. Patient has difficulty in switching from one topic to another or returns to a given topic again and again. Constant repetition of a specific content (theme) is the more severe form of restricted thinking. (AMDP-III, 18)

31. Perseveration: Persistent repetition of words, phrases, sentences, or numbers, to the point of becoming meaningless. Verbigeration, the senseless reiteration of words, is a severe form of perseveration. (AMDP-III, 19)

32. Rumination: Endless preoccupation or incessant concern with somctimes unpleasant thoughts not experienced as alien and usually related to the real situation in the patient's life. Do not rate "Obsessional Thinking" (Item 46) here. (AMDP-III, 20)

33. Pressured Thinking: Driven or kaleidoscopic thinking. Patient feels himself under great stress from disruptive or constantly recurring thoughts-sometimes sensible, sometimes senseless – which seem to tumble over one another. (AMDP-III, 21)

34. Flight of Ideas: Increased number of ideas with a loosening of internal direction or goal. Ideas flow so rapidly that sentences or thoughts are not completed because thinking is continuously interrupted by diverse associations – often clang associations. In contrast to Item 37 ("Incoherence"), the examiner can usually follow the flight of ideas. The acceleration in the flight of ideas is sometimes subjectively perceived as pressured thinking, and should be scored under Item 33. Accelerated thinking without a flight of ideas should be rated under Item 39 ("Accelerated Thinking"). In these latter conditions, the internal connections between ideas are retained. (AMDP-III, 22)

35. Tangential Thinking: Talking past or around the point. Although appearing to understand the question, the patient does not answer directly but brings up another topic or something different in context. Do not rate deliberate avoidance of answers. (AMDP-III, 23)

36. Blocking: Sudden blocks or interruptions in the flow of the thought process without obvious reason. The patient stops in the middle of a sentence, is silent, and then resumes conversation on another topic. (AMDP-III, 24). Blocking occurs in states of clear consciousness and must not be confused with interruptions of thinking due to petit mal. The thought block is experienced by the patient who, however, is not aware of any motive(s) behind the breaks or blocks.

37. Incoherence: Thought and, consequently, speech no longer have understandable connections. What remain are fragmented incomprehensible thoughts, phrases, and sentences arbitrarily thrown together. Thoughts jump from one topic to another. Therefore, incoherent thinking will be unintelligible and cannot be reconstructed. Differs from flight of ideas in that there are no connections whatsoever among the ideas. In the mild form, paralogia, the sentence structure can still remain intact, while in the severe form (paragrammatism) words and syllables are a senseless mixture, as in schizophasia. (AMDP-III, 25). Other symptoms of formal thought disorder frequently resulting from looseness in association can be rated under Item 37.
A. Contamination: Fusion of two or more unrelated items.
B. Condensation: Combination of more or less unrelated widely diverse ideas into one.
C. Substitution: Replacement of familiar concepts with unusual ones.
D. Derailment: Shifting or switching from the main theme to a subsidiary one which intrudes disruptively.
E. Incomplete or desultory thoughts: Odd, eccentric thinking is also rated here.

38. Neologisms: New word or phrase building in which the usual language conventions are not observed and which usually cannot be easily understood. Sometimes the patient may construct or use an artificial language of his own. Includes paralogisms, i.e., sematically unusual use of words. Manneristic speech is rated in Item 102. (AMDP-III, 26)

39. Accelerated Thinking: The speed of thinking and speech is accelerated. Abnormally rapid flow of ideas and verbal output. Often, but not necessarily, associated with Item 34 ("Flight of Ideas") and Item 105 ("Logorrhea").

40. Impaired Abstraction: To be examined by brief testing of the ability to generalize, e.g. naming the conceptual category to which a set of items belong, to perceive commonalities, and to describe the content of abstract ideas.

41. Conceptual Impairment: To be tested by giving the patient several short words or concepts from which a sentence is to be constructed, e.g., auto, traffic light, woman, crossing the street.

42. Impaired Judgment: Disturbance of the critical function. The patient's ability to assess his personal circumstances and abilities accurately and to come to an appropriate judgment of his present situation.

Phobias and Compulsions

43. Suspiciousness: Nondelusional propensity to view the world with anxious uncertainty and mistrust. Inclination to engage in self-referential interpretations greatly affecting the "inner life" and behavior of the patient. A special form is non delusional jealousy. (AMDP-III, 27)

44. Hypochondriasis: Anxious, fearful perception of one's body. Nondelusional misgivings about one's state of health. Objectively unfounded fear of falling ill or being ill. Somatic sensations are perceived fearfully and are given undue attention. Delusional hypochondriasis is differentiated by its absolute conviction of illness. There is some doubt in the non delusional types about the "reality" of the illness. There is more a fear or suspicion of illness. Intermediate forms of hypochondriasis can exist. From fear of cancer, syphilis, or heart disease to mortal dread, e.g., carcinophobia, syphilophobia, cardiophobia, a delusional conviction can develop. Thus, nondelusional hypochondriasis can become delusional over time. (AMDP-III, 28)

45. Phobias: Overwhelming fear which repeatedly occurs in certain situations or in the presence of certain objects – more often than not resulting in the avoidance of the stimulus. Phobias differ from ordinary anxiety in that the compulsive inevitability of the fear is combined with intellectual insight (full, partial, or transient) of its unreasonableness and with the experience of inner resistance against the fear. Phobias can lead to certain behavior – the so-called compulsive avoidance reaction. (AMDP-III, 29)

46. Obsessive Thoughts: Preoccupation with thoughts which persist against one's will and cannot be banished by volitional effort. While obsessive thoughts are not necessarily senseless, their persistence and penetrance must be regarded as senseless and unjustified. Include obsessive ideas, thoughts, images, memories, questions, ruminations, and fears under this category. (AMDP-III, 30)

47. Compulsive Impulses: Persistent drive (urge) to carry out actions against one's will, e.g., the urge to control something, to jump out of a window, to attack somebody, to curse or utter obscene words (coprolalia), to count or calculate (arithmomania). (AMDP-III, 31)

48. Compulsive Actions: Actions persistently carried out against one's will – usually based on compulsive fears or impulses. Frequently a ritual or ceremony is carried out, e.g., handwashing in a precise, uniform, and repetitive manner.

When the ritual has been performed, there is often a "folie de doute," i.e., doubt that the ritual has been performed correctly, thus requiring repetition of the ritual. Repetitiveness, however, can also be seen without such doubt. Pathological laughing or weeping – as release phenomena of inborn expressive movements seen in cerebral disease processes – are not included here. (ADMP-III, 32)

Delusions

There are two types of items under this heading – those concerned with the formal aspects of delusions (Items 49–54) and those concerned with content (Items 55–62).

One can define delusion as a disease-induced misjudgment of reality arising as self-evident to the patient and which is held with unshakable subjective conviction even though it is in contradiction to reality and to the experience of healthy people and the collective beliefs and concepts of mankind. The patient usually feels no need to give reasons for his delusional belief, since, to him, its correctness (reality) is unequivocally certain. Delusions are present in a variety of psychoses and are not specific for schizophrenia.

49. Delusional Mood: The affect which forms the background of the delusional experience. An atmosphere of perplexity and personal involvement in which the world or the self is experienced as strangely changed. The patient very often cannot give details of the content of the changes. The mood consists of unsubstantiated guesses, suppositions, and expectations which, to the healthy person, have no meaning or relationship. There are a variety of moods associated with the subjective belief in the delusional experience. Most often, it is a sense of awe or mystery about the changes in one's self or in the environment. Other common moods are: apprehension, terror, foreboding, fear, suspiciousness, perplexity, and occasionally elation and hope. (AMDP-III, 33)

Example: "Something's in the air," "something's about to happen," or ordinary things in the surroundings take on special meaning.

50. Delusional Perceptions: A normally perceived event (stimulus) is endowed with abnormal significance – usually related to the self – which it does not objectively possess. A delusional perception is actually a delusional misinterpretation of a real perception.

Example: "The tracks in the sky (jet trails) are the fingers of God." "The doctor nodded while shaking my hand which means I have cancer."

Delusional perceptions must be distinguished from Item 63 ("Illusion"). Delusional memories should be coded under Item 25 ("Paramnesia"). (AMDP-III, 34)

51. Sudden Delusional Thoughts: Sudden ("out of the blue") expression of a delusional notion; transient delusional irruptions. (AMDP-III, 35)

52. Delusional Ideas: Isolated, irrational, or delusional thoughts which can emerge singly or in combination; may remain unchanged or can be further elaborated. (AMDP-III, 36)

53. Systematized Delusions: Organized system of delusional ideas. Delusions are assembled into a coherent – albeit irrational – interconnected construct. New delusional perceptions or ideas as well as secondary delusions (delusional elaborations) may be used to produce the system. There are systems in which only the first supposition is clearly delusional. In most cases, systematization is accomplished only after prolonged psychosis and is dependent upon the deterioration of the patient. There are chronically psychotic patients with well-preserved personalities in whom the systematized delusions appear to be the only recognizable symptoms. In paranoia, there are always well-elaborated systematized delusions. The criterion – a recognizable, definite structure with a strong central cohesion – must be strictly met to be rated here. Unsystematized delusions, if also present, are rated in Item 52. (AMDP-III, 37)

54. Delusional Dynamics: The force or intensity of the affective drive which accompanies the delusion. It is possible to estimate the dynamics by the way in which the delusion is reported. There are variations ranging from vivid delusions forcefully narrated and intensely described to monotonous, stiff recitations of usually old delusions reported without affective resonance or productivity. The dynamics are scored "severe" when delusional experiences appear on a vivid or intense affective (sometimes parathymic) background with psychomotor activity and increased drive and when the delusional ideas are flowing rapidly and are marked by intense reactions. The dynamics are scored "mild" or "absent," in long-term, chronic schizophrenics, in whom delusions are often reported in an emotionless, stereotyped way without any recognizable affect (residual delusion). (AMDP-III, 38)

55. Delusions of Reference: The conviction that environmental events or objects have a special meaning for the patient. The patient is convinced that events in the surroundings which, in fact, have nothing to do with him, have a definite significance for him, e.g., that a conversation between others has some reference leading to him or that a casual blink of the eye from a passerby conveys an important message. The patient feels himself to be the focus of observation and attention and even the most insignificant events are sources of extremely important signals for him. Delusions of reference may occur in an isolated form or as the basis or background for other types of delusions, e.g., persecution, grandeur, erotomania. (AMDP-III, 39)

56. Delusions of Persecution: Conviction that persons or organizations are attempting to do harm to the patient. He sees himself as a focus of animosity. He feels that he is threatened, offended, insulted, mocked, or derided by others who are striving to take his money, property, health, or even his life. Querulous (litigious) delusions are a special type of persecutory delusion in which the patient struggles for justice because of some supposed judicial injury. (AMDP-III, 40)

57. Delusions of Jealousy: Delusional conviction of being deceived or betrayed by a loved one. An unsubstantiated or unfounded conviction. (AMDP-III, 41)

58. Delusions of Guilt: Conviction of having failed in one's duty or having wronged others. The patient believes he has failed in his duty to God, to some higher moral code, or has broken the law or a trust. It can be either an imagined guilt or an extreme exaggeration – due to pathological guilt feelings – of actual errors or failures. The patient feels he is evil, inferior, rejected, or unpardonably damned. The guilt may be related to acts of omission, e.g., not taking care of his children, not having sought medical help earlier. Frequently, self-accusations are seen concerning masturbation, perversion, abortion, etc. In rare cases, it may be an existential guilt, e.g., mere existence as a human, in itself, is guilt-laden, having failed in one's task in life – one's individualization. (AMDP-III, 42)

59. Delusions of Impoverishment: Conviction of having lost one's fortune or livelihood. The themes of these delusions center around material loss, e.g., money, clothes, home, sustenance, job. Patient sees himself and his family starving. (AMDP-III, 43)

60. Hypochondriacal Delusions: Conviction of improbable or impossible physical illness. The patient is convinced that his health is threatened, that he is chronically ill, or that he is about to die. The content can also be concerned with specific illnesses, e.g., cancer, syphilis, multiple sclerosis, progressive paralysis, brain atrophy, mental illness. Nihilistic delusions are rated here.

Example: "My bowels are completely blocked" (despite the fact that he defecates regularly). "My sex organs are dead and will not function again." "I'm dead."

Hypochondriacal delusions may appear to be like coenesthetic hallucinations seen in schizophrenia. The abnormal bodily sensations of the depressive, however, do not have the character of "having been caused by outside forces," so often seen in schizophrenic hypochondriacal delusions. The bizarre character of the complaints reported, the parathymia as well as the general affective state and the appearance of associated disturbances of the ego usually make it possible to differentiate schizophrenic hypochondriacal delusions from depressive ones. The bizarre character of hypochondriacal delusions of the schizophrenic are exemplified by the following examples: "Every night they dry up my lungs." "Every time I eat, they turn my entrails to ashes." "My brain has been softened and in its place is a lake of pus." (AMDP-III, 44)

61. Delusions of Grandeur: Expansive or fantastic claims of one's abilities or position. The patient is convinced that he is superior to all other people by virtue of his talents, power, abilities, wealth, etc. He believes himself to be most powerful, the ruler of the world, God, or an envoy of God. There may be delusions of distinguished birth or having made great inventions. Religious delusions are rated here. The patient may believe he has been sent by or has some special relation with God or has been given a sacred mission to perform in the world. (AMDP-III, 45)

62. Other Delusions: Delusional themes not categorized above should be specified and scored here. (AMDP-III, 46)

Disorders of Perception

63. Illusions: Distortion of a real perception. Falsified actual perceptions, the presence of a real object (percept) differentiates an illusion from a hallucination.

Example: At night, the frightened child perceived a poorly lit bush to be a threatening figure. (AMDP-III, 47)

Remarks on Hallucinations – Hallucinations are perceptual experiences without a corresponding stimulus in the environment. One can hallucinate in all sense modalities and frequently in more than one. The judgment of reality is more or less narrowed or suspended.

64. Verbal (Phonemic) Hallucinations: Perception of human voices without external stimuli. Voices of humanoids are also included, e.g., God, Satan, spacemen, robots, leprechauns. There are different degrees of clarity and substance to the voices. The voices may speak directly to the patient, or may be experienced (overheard) as conversations between third persons. Thoughts heard aloud by the patient (echo de pense) should be encoded here. It is sometimes difficult to differentiate phonemes from Item 73 ("Thought Insertion"). (AMDP-III, 48)

65. Other Auditory Hallucinations: Includes all nonphonemic auditory hallucinations, e.g., animals, birds, trees, inanimate objects, akousma. (AMDP-III, 49)

66. Visual Hallucinations: Visual perceptions without corresponding external stimuli. Range from simple optical phenomena (photomes) to elaborate scenes, e.g., "Everything is brillantly colored," "Like in the movies," "Like a big painting." (AMDP-III, 50)

67. Bodily Hallucinations (Coenesthetic): Unfounded tactile and somatic perceptions including touch, kinesthesic, pain, pressure, and thermic phenomena. Many such hallucinations have the character of being produced by external forces, e.g., the patient feels he is being abused sexually by electricity or "rays." Rather common in geriatric patients are the skin sensations associated with delusions of infestation. It is not always easy to differentiate bodily hallucinations from other delusional experiences, especially when perceptions of space and motion as well as of internal organs are involved. (AMDP-III, 51)

68. Olfactory or Gustatory Hallucinations: Hallucinations in these sense modalities often occur together, alternate, or merge with one another. (AMDP-III, 52)

According to Jaspers (15), ego disorders include disturbances in experiencing the self as "one" in a moment of time (ego-integrity), as one in the course of time (ego-identity), and as distinct from the environment (ego-boundary). Item 70 ("Depersonalization") is an impairment of ego-world boundaries. Items 71 ("Thought Broadcasting"), 72 ("Thought Withdrawal"), 73 ("Thought Insertion"), and 74 ("Other Feelings of Alien Influence") are all disturbances of ego integrity.

69. Derealization: The experience of one's environment being unreal, strange, or otherwise changed. To the patient, the world appears unfamiliar, peculiar, ghostly, or somehow changed. These feelings of estrangement can be part of a delusional mood. Changes in time perception are included here, as is a reduced vividness of sensory experiences, e.g., in depression. (AMDP-III, 53)

70. Depersonalization: Disturbances of the unity (oneness) of the self in the present or in one's identity in the course of illness. The experience of one's self being unreal, detached, strange, changed, or unidentifiable.

These ego disturbances can be fleeting or persistent. A disturbance of ego-identity over the course of time is present when the patient perceives himself as somebody different than he was at an earlier time and questions whether it was him or someone else. He does not know anymore who has experienced his past.

Example: Patient proclaims himself Professor of Veterinary Medicine and Director of the Institution, and states he is here to produce hebephrenia. Another male patient discovers he has become a woman (delusional sex transformation).

Transformation delusions, e.g., becoming an animal (lycanthropy) are also included here.

Delusional disturbances of ego-awareness should be differentiated from the so-called *"Doppelganger"* experience or autoscopy – the phenomenon in which the person perceives his own form from outside himself. The nucleus of the ego remains intact when these phenomena occur. Through certain partial drives in the personality gaining autonomy, splitting and doubling experiences can occur. These disturbances, however, should be differentiated from the so-called multiple personality. In this unusual phenomenon, the patient, for a period of time, experiences and declares himself to be another person and has no memory of the earlier person. Thus, there is a succession of different personalities each of which, however, has a unified ego-consciousness, whereas in the true disturbance of ego-awareness the different personalities are simultaneously experienced and act side by side. Misidentification of his own person – when there is preserved ego consciousness – should be rated in Item 9 ("Disturbances of Self-Orientation"). Transitivism and appersonalization are rated here. (AMDP-III, 54)

71. Thought Broadcasting: The experience that one's thoughts are not exclusively one's own, but are shared by others. The patient complains that "People know what I think. Everybody knows what goes on in my head." Audible thoughts, a kind of broadcasting in which the patient believes his thoughts are heard by others, are rated here. (AMDP-III, 55)

72. Thought Withdrawal: The experience that thoughts are being removed or pulled out of one's mind. "Thought Withdrawal" should be differentiated from Item 36, "Blocking." (AMDP-III, 56)

73. Thought Insertion: Thoughts, images, etc. are externally introduced into one's mind and influence, direct, or impel behavior.

Example: "They've hypnotized thoughts into my head which aren't mine." (AMDP-III, 57)

74. Other Feelings of Alien Influence: Similar to the feeling that one's thoughts are directed by outside forces, the patient believes that other aspects of his being (feelings, strivings, will, behavior) are being influenced from outside. As a consequence, the patient must say something peculiar, scream, roar, behave in a peculiar way, attack someone, bluster, etc.

Example: "It's not me screaming, it's somebody else. The rays are directing my mouth and speech muscles. The voices scream out of me. I myself do not roar."

Just as in thought insertion, this is also a morbid change in one's action awareness. [15] (AMDP-III, 58)

Disturbance of Affect

75. Perplexity: Mood of uncertainty or puzzlement. The patient is no longer sure of himself, his situation, his surroundings, or his future. He experiences all this subjectively. He cannot understand what is happening to him, what he is supposed to think, plan, or do. He is unable to come to grips with events or provide himself an overview of them. Objective manifestations of perplexity are a puzzled, strange, or anxiously uncertain facial expression; sometimes there is restlessness or hesitant immobility, indecisiveness, searching behavior, and phrases like "What's the matter? Where am I? What's happening? I dont' know. I don't understand!" Perplexity can be found in various conditions, e.g., delusions and confusional states, during emergence from states of disturbed consciousness like anesthesia, and even in cases of severe memory disturbance. (AMDP-III, 59)

76. Feeling of Loss of Feeling: Feeling that one has lost the ability for emotional resonance; loss or absence of feeling, feeling of emotional emptiness, feeling that one's emotions are "dead."

Example: "I feel dead inside. I'm not able to feel anything at all. It's empty and dead within me. I don't feel pleasure or sadness or excitement – everything is without feeling." (AMDP-III, 60)

77. Blunted Affect: Observed decrease in emotional responsiveness, e.g., meager feelings, emotional indifference, lack of concern, loss of interest. If the patient complains about the indifference, Item 76 ("Feeling of Loss of Feeling") must be encoded also. (AMDP-III, 61)

78. Felt Loss of Vitality: Depression of general bodily feelings subjectively experienced by the patient. Disturbance in the underlying feeling of being alive. Loss or reduction in energy, liveliness, and vigor. Also included are the general feelings of fatigue, weakness, bodily discomfort, and lack of "pep" or animation.

Example: "It's all so difficult. I have no bounce. I'm weighed down and am so tired."

Strong, localized disturbances, e.g., headache, feeling of fullness (bloat), pressure (tightness) in the chest, and muscle weakness in specific areas are not included here. They should be rated under the appropriate items of "Part 5 – Somatic Signs." (AMDP-III, 62)

79. Depressed Mood: Negatively tinged affective state characterized by lowered mood and experienced as sadness. It must be present during the evaluation or within the prescribed rating period. Depression covers a wide spectrum of feelings from sadness, uneasiness, loss of pleasure, dullness, dejectedness, and loss of interest to feelings of grief, sorrow, despair, helplessness, and extreme, indescribable inner torment. The expressions of depressive symptomatology vary: crying, looking sad, downcast, or in despair, and looking as though in pain or torment are all expressions of depression. (AMDP-III, 63)

80. Hopelessness: Despondent, despairing, pessimistic mood with lack of positive expectations. (AMDP-III, 64)

81. Anxiety: Fearfulness or apprehensive feelings without specification or objective basis. The symptom should be explored explicitly with the patient and the rating should be based on the subjective experience and not just on the expression and behavior of the patient. (AMDP-III, 65)

82. Euphoria: Heightened mood or elevated sense of well-being. Excessive cheerfulness or serenity reaching to feelings of elation and ecstasy. (AMDP-III, 66)

83. Dysphoria: A morose, sullen, dissatisfied mood. Ill-humored, crabby, nagging, discordant attitude. (AMDP-III, 67)

84. Irritability: Undercurrent of anger or aggressiveness. The examiner can sense the imminence of aggressively tinged, affective outbursts even when the patient exhibits a seemingly calm exterior (tense calm). (AMDP-III, 68)

85. Inner Restlessness: Complaints or feelings of psychic unrest. The patient complains spontaneously – or in response to questions – that he is stirred by and suffers from agitation and tension. Do not include Item 100 ("Motor Restlessness") here. Inner restlessness is frequently associated with depressive, fearful, hopeless, and despondent feelings and with manic states, delusional mood, and delusional states with various content. (AMDP-III, 69)

86. Complaintativeness: Expressions of pain and grief through words, mimicry, and gesture. Wailing, weeping, sighing, groaning, and other similar phenomena are seen. Lamentation – loud and repetitive complaints expressed in a morose way – is also rated here. (AMDP-III, 70)

87. Feelings of Inadequacy: Imagined lessened capacity. Nondelusional feeling that one is incompetent, incapable, clumsy, awkward, indecisive, dumb, ignorant, dowdy, etc. The feeling or pronounced loss of self-esteem should be scored "Severe." (AMDP-III, 71)

88. Exaggerated Self-esteem: Heightened self-confidence. High opinion of one's abilities and strengths. Although nondelusional, the patient believes himself to be very unusual, e.g., very smart, very strong, very competent, very talented, very powerful, very rich, etc. (AMDP-III, 72)

89. Feelings of Guilt: Exaggerated remorse for past behavior, thoughts, or wishes which, in the patient's eyes, go against moral or religious tenets. Delusions of guilt are encoded under Item 58. (AMDP-III, 73)

90. Feelings of Impoverishment: Nondelusional feeling that one does not have the means to sustain one's livelihood. Delusional impoverishment is encoded in Item 59. (AMDP-III, 74)

91. Ambivalence: Coexisting, contradicting conscious feelings which the patient experiences simultaneously and most often as harassing.

Example: Love and hate for a particular person at the same time.

Avoid confusion with Item 75 ("Perplexity") and Item 107 ("Indecisiveness"). (AMDP-III, 75)

92. Parathymia: Paradoxical affect. Inappropriate emotional expression or response to a situation.

Example: A patient describes how he was tormented the night before and, while doing so, is laughing. Another patient is delighted with a gift, yet is lamenting its receipt at the same time (paramimia). (AMDP-III, 76)

93. Affective Lability: Rapid changes in affect. Increases in affective variability in which an affect persists for only a very short period and shows many ups and downs. Take into consideration native temperament or cultural tradition. (AMDP-III, 77)

94. Affective Incontinence: Lack or loss of emotional control. Rash outbursts of affect which are uncontrolled and often of great intensity. (AMDP-III, 78)

95. Affective Rigidity: Reduction or loss of emotional modulation. The patient persists, without modulation or oscillation, in certain moods or affects regardless of the external situation. If there is still a degree of modulation in the existing affect, rate "mild." If more than one affect suddenly emerges, rate this item "absent." (AMDP-III, 79)

Drive is essentially independent of will. It is the animating (energizing) force that is the impetus behind the tempo, intensity, and endurance of all psychological performance. Drive is recognized by the animation, verve, initiative, alertness, energy, or enterprise exhibited by the individual. Drive is primarily recognized in expressive, psychomotor behavior.

96. Lack of Drive: Deficient energy or initiative. Subjectively reported by the patient or observed by the interviewer as sparse motor behavior and/or decreased initiation of conversation. An example is the quiet, passive patient who cannot be prompted into conversation and who seems to be submerged within himself. In "Stupor" (Item 98), there is a loss of motoric activity with a maximum loss of drive. (AMDP-III, 80)

97. Inhibition of Drive: In contrast to lack of drive, inhibition does not refer to the diminution of energy and initiative of the patient, but rather to a slowing down (Braking) of drive. The patient's efforts to overcome the inhibition can be quite obvious to the interviewer. Inhibition can be seen in psychomotor activity, in perceptual experience, and in thought processing. The patient tries to overcome the inhibition, but cannot seem to brighten up; he stops trying, then tries to pull himself together again, etc. (AMDP-III, 81)

98. Stuporous: The most important hallmarks of stupor are the lack of motility and the loss of reactivity without neurological abnormalities – in contrast to coma. The patient does not move or is very slowed down in movement. Speech is sparse or absent. There is little or no response to being called or to other approaches. The patient gives no understandable indications of his mental processes and one can no longer make contact with him.

99. Increased Drive: Increase in activity and initiative as compared to the usual activity level. The behavior usually remains organized and purposeful. (AMDP-III, 82)

100. Motor Restlessness: Aimless and purposeless motor activity which can increase to frenzy. The patient is continually in motion, running around (motor restlessness with locomotion) or moving his limbs while remaining in place. Restlessness can also be circumscribed, e.g., scratching, handwringing, ticlike movements. (AMDP-III, 83)

101. Parakinesia: Qualitatively abnormal, complex movements which often affect gestures, facial expressions, or speech. Motor stereotypy involves a tendency to repeat – in exactly the same form and often for a long time–speech or motoric expressions. In contrast to Item 31 ("Perseveration"), the connection to words and/or gestures previously used in the conversation cannot be recognized. Verbigeration, the stereotypy of words, is also rated here. Score catalepsy, waxy flexibility, automatic behaviors, automatic obedience, and echo symptoms here. The patient carries out automatic acts which he does not perceive as intentional and automatically follows commands. When the stimulus for such behavior is mainly by example and the movements of the patient consist of imitation, it is called echopraxia. When there is an imitation of words or sentences, it is called echolalia. (AMDP-III, 84)

102. Mannerisms: Natural movements and behavior (gestures, facial expression, speech) become exaggerated, distorted, posed, and baroque – often in a pronounced playful fashion. Manneristic behavior also refers to unnatural, pompous, boastful (in the sense of bombastic), studied, affected and artificial, cramped, stylistic, showy, and bizarre behavior. Compared with his group standards, a manneristic patient behaves in an extraordinarily conspicuous fashion in speech, movement, or dress. (AMDP-III, 85)

103. Histrionics: Theatricality. The patient gives the impression that he is exaggerating his situation, difficulties, and disturbances. His behavior often appears markedly demonstrative. (AMDP-III, 86)

104. Mutism: Parsimonious speech or the absence of speech for psychological reasons. The patient generally no longer speaks or whispers only very few words or syllables. Mutism can be the result of drive deficiency, inhibition, or blocking. It may also be an active, negativistic refusal to make verbal contact. (AMDP-III, 87)

105. Logorrhea: Voluble speech. Speaking with unquenchable pressure and too excessively for understanding. Depending on its tempo, clarity, internal cohesiveness, and logical or meaningful connections, logorrhea can be quite comprehensible or not at all comprehensible to the interviewer. (AMDP-III, 88)

106. Negativism: The patient will not do immediately or at all what one expects or requires of him (passive negativism) or he does the opposite (active negativism).

107. Indecisiveness: The patient is not able to make a decision within a reasonable period of time. Vacillation.

Part 4 – Psychopathological Symptoms

This section consists of a catalogue of symptoms which are much more directed toward the geriatric patient than was the case in Part 3. As such, this section has less correspondence to the AMDP-III. Nevertheless, some 24% of the symptoms listed in this section are common to both the AGP and the AMDP-III.

108. Psychoorganic Syndrome: A three-part item. This syndrome is evaluated in toto, i.e., globally (Items 108–111), and in particular, i.e., by functional brain areas (Items 112–134).

If the entire syndrome is absent, circle "O" beside the heading; leave the entire section blank and proceed to "Circadian Disturbances."

A. Site: One entry only. The choices are:

Localized: In addition to the change in drive (increase or decrease) and disturbance of affect, there is a disturbance of a *single* drive, e.g., bulimia, impulsive sexual behavior.

Diffuse: Besides the existence of disturbances of memory, attention, and poverty of thought, it is characterized by an affect disturbance manifested as aspontaneity and blunting to the point of apathy. Also there are frequent definite episodes of restlessness.

B. Severity: Immediate verification for the rating of this pragmatic clinical scale can be obtained by using brief and uniform tests for organic disturbance in the psychogeriatric patient. Before making a decision on the severity of organic disturbance, however, it is necessary to assess for severity of temporospatial disorientation.

Mild (MI): No demonstrable temporospatial disorientation as indicated by the presence of one or more significant disturbances of basic intellectual functions, e.g., memory, perceptions, attention, concentration, apperception. Rating this item can raise the question of whether a specific loss, e.g., memory, is or is not "normal" or "age appropriate." To avoid confusion, use the following uniform rule: Evaluate the pathology of each demonstrable loss independent of the age at which it occurs.

Moderate (MO): Partial temporospatial disorientation, i.e., unequivocal loss in certain aspects of space/time orientation with retention of unimpaired orientation in at least one element in the presence of one or more significant disturbances of basic intellectual functions, e.g., memory, perception, concentration, apperception.

Severe (SV): Corresponds to the concept of dementia. Total temporospatial disorientation, i.e., practically none of the elements of space/time orientation are retained in the presence of one or more significant disturbances of basic intellectual functions.

C. Duration: The time elapsed (time span) since the first appearance of significant organic loss – taking into account all available information.

Note: The category "Global Performance Disturbances" must be completed in every case. Detailed assessment of the subsequent category "Localized Brain Dysfunction" is optional.

Global Performance Disturbances

If no disturbances are present in this category, i.e., Items 109–111, circle "O"; leave the items blank and proceed to next category – "Localized Brain Dysfunction."

109. Aphasia: Disturbance of receptive or expressive speech on the basis of a central dysfunction despite unimpaired hearing and/or intact vocal apparatus.

110. Agnosia: Inability to recognize sensory input as a consequence of central disturbance despite an intact functional capability of the involved sense organ. Agnosia is usually limited to one sensory field, e.g., sight, taste. Stereoagnosia is the inability of the patient to identify through touch an object which he can recognize by sight.

111. Apraxia: Inability to carry out dexterous, purposeful, and appropriate movements. Inability to move volitionally and purposefully parts of one's body despite intact motor apparatus.

Localized Brain Dysfunctions:

Circle "O" if no disturbances are present under this major rubric, i.e., Items 112–134; leave items blank and proceed to the category "Circadian Disturbances."

Fronto parietal Disturbances

Circle "O" if none of the subsumed items (112–116) are present.

112. Frontal Apraxia: Loss of static and locomotor function, e.g., astasia-abasia, occasionally with a grotesque, almost comic, incoordination in walking *(Witzelsucht der Beine).*

113. Facial Apraxia: Bucco-linguo-facial apraxia. Tested by the patient sticking out the tongue, showing the teeth, opening the mouth, pursing the lips, and closing the eyes.

114. Prefrontal Impulse Syndrome: Characterized by a lack of drive, aspontaneity, indifference, slowness, dynamic aphasia (adynamic speech). When seen with preserved reactivity, it is called frontal akinesia.

115. Frontobasal Impulse Syndrome: Characterized by a lack of inhibition, jocularity, lack of concern, and optimism. Disturbances of smell are frequent here.

116. Motor Aphasia: As a consequence of a central motor dysfunction, voluntary expressive speech is a partial or total impossibility despite preserved receptive speech. The patient utters only mutilated words or disconnected syllables.

Occipital Disturbances

If Items 117–122 are "absent," circle "O" and proceed to "Parieto-occipital Disturbance." Disturbances of color perception (Items 117–119) are concerned with three tests or impaired color perception.

117. Inability to Recognize a Color: A color is presented and the patient is asked "Is this ________ (red, blue, etc.)?"

118. Inability to Name a Color: A color is presented and the patient is asked to name it.

119. Inability to Visualize a Color: Patient is asked "What is the color of a ________ (banana, tomato, etc.)?"

120. Visual Agnosia: Inability to interpret the significance of perceptions (mind-blindness). Object, e.g., key, pencil, comb, are not recognized or are named as such by sight alone – although they can be recognized through touch. Further, failure on the basis of memory to recognize or describe shapes, persons, colors, etc.

121. Prosopagnosia: Impaired or distorted recognition of faces and their expressive features.

122. Dysmorphopsia: Distorted perception of objects despite unimpaired vision. The patient frequently perceives objects as larger, smaller, or tilted.

Parieto-occipital Disturbances

If Items 123–132 are "absent," circle "O" and proceed to "Temporal Disturbances."

123. Stereoagnosia: Tactile agnosia. Inability to identify objects by touch despite intact sensation.

Example: With eyes closed, inability to recognize a familiar object placed in one's hand, e.g., key, spoon, pencil, or safety pin.

124. Somatagnosia: Disturbance of the body image. Inability to identify the body or its parts or to orient oneself to the body. Inability to point out – on one's own body as well as another's – the nose, ear, eye, elbow, foot, knee, etc.; i.e., a disturbance of right/left differentiation not only on one's own body but on the examiner's body and in the surroundings. This symptom should only be scored if, through testing, a disturbance in vertical orientation has been excluded and it is patently clear that the disturbance of right/left orientation is actually present in the patient.

125. Anosognosia: Nonrecognition and disregard of a somatic dysfunction – above all, denial of hemiplagia, especially left-sided hemiplegia or damage to the nondominant hemisphere. The paralyzed side is totally ignored or nor longer recognized as one's own, e.g., in confusion, the patient may grasp his own paralyzed arm with his healthy hand instead of the proferred arm of the examiner.

126. Conduction Aphasia: Inability to repeat dictated speech as presented. Isolated disturbances often combined with paraphasia and paragraphia. To examine, present patient with short sentences – gradually increasing their length – and have the patient repeat them word for word.

127. Alexia: Reading disturbances. Diminution of reading ability; letter and/or word blindness, Inability to read written material despite intact vision.

128. Agraphia: Writing disturbance. Inability to write despite intact intelligence and motor function of the arm and hand. A consequence of damage in a specific central region where the necessary function capacities are formed.

129. Acalculia: Inability to carry out simple calculations, although the patient should be able to perform on the basis of previous education and training.

130. Ideomotor Apraxia: Inability to carry out specific, simple task on command. Each hand should be tested separately, e.g., winking, making a fist, combing one's hair, biting an apple, throwing a ball, using a key.

131. Ideational Apraxia: Inability to carry out familiar, complex activities of everyday life, e.g., telephoning, making coffee, setting out dishes, lighting a cigarette, dressing and undressing. Kleist's test for apraxia may be used here, i.e., tear a sheet of paper in half, roll it up with one hand, and then use the other hand to snatch it away. Demonstrate and have the patient imitate the procedure with each hand.

132. Constructional Apraxia: Inability to construct two- and especially three dimensional spatial representations. Is seen in the inability to draw or construct geometric figures correctly, e.g., failure to reproduce spontaneously or copy from a picture, objects such as a circle, rectangle, triangle, man, house, flower, bicycle, and cube. Inability to copy or construct such figures with the help of matches. Also rated here are such inabilities as tieing a tie or shoelaces, and putting on or taking off a jacket.

Temporal Disturbances

If Items 133–134 are "absent," circle "O" and proceed to "Circadian Disturbances."

133. Amnestic Aphasia (Nominal Aphasia): Inability to reproduce the names of objects, qualities, or conditions. May be recognized, however, with hints. Above all, it is the inaccessibility of the noun. The patient cannot name the object, e.g., key, clock, or pencil, but can describe, in detail, its use. For example, on being shown a pencil the patient may exclaim, "That's to write with."

134. Sensory Aphasia: Loss of speech comprehension (receptive speech) with intact motor speech. It results in jumbled speech, incorrectly used words, mutilations, omissions, paraphasia, word salad, jargon, etc. In contrast to motor aphasia, the marked production of speech is characteristic.

Circadian Disturbances

Oscillations in condition or behavior of the patient during a 24-hour period. Seasonal oscillations should not be included here.

135. Worse in the Morning: Condition is worse between 12 midnight and 12 noon. (AMDP-III, 89)

136. Worse in the Evening: Condition is worse between 12 noon and 12 midnight. (AMDP-III, (90)

137. Better in the Evening: Distinct improvement of condition in the evening. Do not score if improvement is only relative when compared with morning low. (AMDP-III, 91)

138. Nighttime Exacerbation: Eruption or significant increase in psychopathological phenomena during the night hours.

139. Symptom Alternation: Changes in contrasting symptoms within a 24-hour period (aggressiveness to timidity, happiness to sadness).

Disturbances of Sleep and Vigilance

140. Difficulty Falling Asleep (Early Insomnia): The time required to fall asleep is experienced by the patient as extended, disturbed, or troubled. (AMDP-III, 101)

141. Interrupted Sleep (Middle Insomnia): A single interruption with quick return to sleep is scored "mild." Frequent interruptions with considerable reduction in sleep are scored "severe." Interruptions for urination are not included here. (AMDP-III, 102)

142. Early Waking (Late Insomnia): Distinct change (advancement) in the usual waking time without the ability to go back to sleep. (AMDP-III, 104)

143. Prolonged Sleep: Lengthening of the duration of sleep within a 24-hour period in comparison to premorbid norm.

144. Shortened Sleep: Reduction or shortening in the amount of sleep required in comparison to premorbid norm. Experienced by the patient as a decreased need for sleep. (AMDP-III, 103)

145, 146. Nighttime Restlessness/Nighttime Confusion: These two symptoms are separated since restlessness and agitation without confusion and, conversely, confusion without restlessness and agitation can occur. As a rule, however, both symptoms occur together and can be so rated by appropriate entries for each symptom.

147. Daytime Drowsiness: Feelings of sleepiness or weariness which do not affect performance are scored "mild"; actually falling asleep during the day is scored "severe." (AMDP-III, 105)

148. Day-Night Rhythm Reversal: Tendency to sleep during the day and to remain awake at night. The tendency can be only suggestive or very pronounced and can be so rated in the item as "mild" to "severe."

149. Increased Dreaming: The patient reports increased dream or nightmare activity compared with previous levels.

Disturbances of Social Behavior

150. Social Withdrawal: Decreased social contact. Judge by the accessibility of the patient in conversation or by the ability to communicate on the ward and/or with people outside the clinic. (AMDP-III, 92)

151. Excessive Social Contact: Markedly increased social contact in comparison with earlier behavior. The patient turns toward many people with an almost total loss of psychological distance, e.g., behavior which is sticky, clinging, superficial, machinating, stifling, or querulous. (AMDP-III, 93)

152. Aggressiveness: Aggressive tendencies: refers to the inclination for violence (verbal or physical) either in attacking other or in defending self. Aggressive acts: refers to physical assault on persons or surroundings. Both tendencies and acts may be rated according to severity. (AMDP-III, 94)

153. Suicidal Tendencies: Suicidal intentions, plans, death wishes, preparations, or attempts. Each of these can be rated from "mild" to "severe." (AMDP-III, 95)

154. Self-mutilation: Includes non-life-threatening, self-inflicted damage, e.g., banging the head against a wall, scratching or cutting the skin, pricking with a needle, plucking out hair (trichotillomania). (AMDP-III, 96)

155. Lack of Feeling Ill: The patient denies, spontaneously or upon questioning, that he feels ill. The differentiation between feeling ill psychologically or physically is not relevant. (AMDP-III, 97)

156. Lack of Insight: The patient is unable to recognize as morbid those experiences or acts which the doctor has judged to be due to disease. (AMDP-III, 98)

157. Uncooperativeness: Negative or oppositional behavior. Resistance against or refusal of various therapeutic measures and/or against admission to the hospital. (AMDP-III, 99)

158. Dissimulation: The patient exhibits a conscious tendency to conceal or suppress his illness or an individual symptom of the illness.

159. Self-neglect: In addition to one's needs, includes neglect of personal hygiene, of dress, and of housekeeping tasks. A deterioration in the physical condition and personal appearance of the patient should be observed and not anticipated from the patient's history.

160. Refusal of Nourishment: Partial or total refusal to eat or drink.

161. Decreased Libido: Reduction in or loss of sexual appetite as compared with the patient's usual libidinal level. (AMDP-III, 109)

162. Increased Libido: Increase in or an exaggeration of sexual appetite in comparison to usual libidinal level.

Social and Nursing Needs

The examiner should assess the social and nursing needs after reviewing all available information. All 14 items subsumed under this rubric (163–176) should be rated systematically on the basis of whether the patient can carry out a range of routine activities almost independently ("mild"), with some help ("moderate"), or is almost completely or completely dependent ("severe"). Comparable assessments are based on disturbances in the somatic and nursing areas. Each behavioral restriction should be determined on the same criteria whether the roots are psychological (depression, dementia) or somatic (paralysis).

163. Financial Needs: If the patient has difficulty in handling financial affairs which do not result in nonpayment of regular budget items, e.g., rent and utilities, rate "mild." If payment are tardy or lapsed, rate "moderate." "Severe" financial needs exist when the level of destitution requires assistance from or dependence upon public social welfare agencies.

164. Housekeeping: Inability to carry out routine household tasks, e.g., dusting, cleaning, making beds.

165. Continuing Medical Care: Need for drugs, medical, and nursing care.

166. Walking: Gait disturbances; difficulty in climbing or descending stairs.

167. Dressing Oneself: Inability to dress/undress or inadequacy of dress, e.g., not warm enough.

168. Personal Hygiene: Difficulties in bathing, shaving, washing, etc.

169. Eating: Difficulties with selecting, preparing, or eating appropriate food.

170. Leisure Activities: Reduced participation in or lack of accessibility to free-time activities.

171. Ability to Use Public Transportation: All restrictions should be assessed, whether they are due to disorientation or physical disability, e.g., a problem in entering or exiting vehicles or buildings.

172. Chewing Disturbance: A need created by deficiency of dentition, e.g., poorly fitted dentures ("mild") to missing prothesis ("severe").

173. Bedridden: Rate degree of restriction or confinement to bed.

174. Urinary Incontinence: Rate the frequency of incontinence.

175. Fecal Incontinence: As in Item 174.

176. Smearing: Includes smearing feces on one's self or on the surroundings.

Reliability of Information

After completing Part 4 Psychopathological Symptoms," the interviewer rates the reliability of the information upon which the assessments are based, i.e., the degree of certainty concerning the validity of the information.

0 = Reliable
1 = Minor inconsistencies or contradictions
2 = Some questionable information, but essentially reliable
3 = Significant amount of unreliable information
4 = Unacceptable degree of reliability

Additional Examinations

Record whether ancillary examinations have been performed by circling the appropriate "Y" (Yes). If no other examinations have been performed, circle "O" and leave all subsumed items blank.

EKG	– Electrocardiography
EEG	– Electroencephalography
Echoencephalography	
CAT	– Computerized axial tomography
Scintiscan	
Dopplersonography	
Angiography	
ENG	– Electronystagmography
LP	– Lumbar puncture
PEG	– Pneumoencephalography
EMG	– Electromyography
Psych. Tests	– Psychological tests
RCBF	– Regional cerebral blood flow
Other (Specify)	

Part 5 – Somatic Signs

This section is intended to document, in a relatively global manner, the geriatric and other somatic (physical) diseases of the patient. The assessment of intensity often has to be based on the subjective clinical impression of the examiner, since evidence upon which to judge severity is not available in every case. Part 5 is organized in three sections:

1. A global judgment of the patient's general state of health
2. An assessment of general somatic disorders
3. An assessment of neurological disorders

The global judgment of general health should reflect an estimation of all somatic disturbances given the practical limitations of the examination. The symptoms listed in section 2 are global and are meant to evaluate the functional deficit of individual organ systems without making syndromal, nosological, or causal determination. The third section, "Neurological Disturbances," on the contrary, is a very detail review of neurological signs which, however, does not represent a systematic neurological assessment – rather it is a framework to be combined by and elaborated upon through a specific neurological examination.

The AGP Somatic Signs differ from the AMDP-III Somatic Signs since they involve a much more thorough review of somatic and neurological disturbances. Nevertheless, a little under 30% of the symptoms are common to both. (Some AMDP-III, Part 5 symptoms are contained in AGP Part 4 as well as AGP Part 5.)

Global State of Health

1. Global State of Health: As far as possible, psychogenic deficit should be separated from somatogenic deficit. The examiner, therefore, must judge for himself, first, the totality of individual findings, and then, their severity in terms of their consequences for the total organism. Finally, the examiner must evolve a single subjective global impression of the patient's infirmity. On this latter point, the patient's level of disability and his compensatory capacity should be considered as well as the objective findings. The judgment is based not only on pathological processes per se, but also on impairment of somatic efficiency resulting from the physiological aging process.

The global state of health is rated as follows:

Good: No serious single finding, only mild age-appropriate disturbances which merely hamper the somatic efficiency of the patient minimally or not at all.
Fair: One or, more often, several disease processes are diagnosed which in toto, however, do not result in serious functional disturbance. Mild to moderate insufficiencies under exertion which can be therapeutically compensated for are included here, e.g., cardiac insufficiency compensated with digitalis, treatable asthma without functional damage.
Poor: The patient's total functioning is markedly damaged on the basis of several disease processes. The damage may be present even at rest or be seen as a serious disturbance during the least exertion, e.g., liver cirrhosis, decompensated cardiac insufficiency, bronchial asthma with frequent occurrences of status asthmaticus.

Somatic Disorders

Cardiovascular Disorders

All disturbances of the cardiovascular system in which depletion of the oxygen supply has resulted are documented here. If Items 2–5 are "absent," circle "O" and proceed to "Respiratory Disorders" (Item 6).

2. Cardiac Insufficiency: Defined as the inability of the organ to transport all available venous blood into the arterial system and thus satisfy the requirements of peripheral circulation. Consequences thus range from congestion to drop in blood volume/minute.

Mild: No symptoms while at rest; however, there is nycturia, mild daytime edema with movement, or dyspnea only under increased physical stress with proportional tachycardia.

Moderate: Dyspnea already seen under a neglible degree of bodily activity; restriction of efficiency, edema in the legs which persists at rest, nycturia.

Severe: Corresponds to decompensated cardiac insufficiency with dyspnea at rest, congestive symptoms, and incapacitation even without exertion in which the patient is almost totally bedridden.

3. Dysrhythmia: All forms of rhythmic disturbances are rated globally. Differentiation between impulse and conduction disturbances is not necessary.

4. Hypertension: Persistent increases of mean arterial blood pressure which exceed the norm should be encoded. Independent of age, diastolic presssure of more than 90 mmHg is to be considered elevated, while depending upon age, an upper limit of systolic pressure is assumed to be 140–160 mmHg. According to WHO, any systolic pressure over 160 mmHg and any diastolic pressure over 95 mmHg are diagnostic of hypertension. The rating of severity is based on the Keith-Wagener criteria.[1]

Mild (K-W I): Includes patients with a mild, mostly labile, hypertension characterized especially by transient increases in blood pressure without systemic complications or eye-

[1] K-W I = No or negligible eyeground change
K-W II = Advanced vascular changes
K-W III = Retinal bleeding
K-W IV = Retinal bleeding accompanied by papilledema

ground changes. Resting blood pressure in these patients lies at or slightly above the upper limit of the normal range.

Moderate (K-W II): Patients with significant subjective complaints, e.g., anginal pain, dyspnea, headache, dizziness, dry mouth belong here. Substantial organic changes are almost never clinically demonstrable. Eyeground changes = K-W I or II. Diastolic blood pressure ranges between 110 and 125 mmHg.

Severe (K-W III): Patients as a rule manifest clinical systemic complications, e.g., eyeground changes. Diastolic blood pressure ranges between 125 and 140 mmHg.

K-W IV Level: Identical with a malignant phase. This group includes patients with markedly increased diastolic blood pressure, progressive overall insufficiency, or papilledema.

5. *Other Disturbances:* Specify any disturbances not subsumed under preceding items.

Respiratory Disorders

6. *Respiratory Disorders:* Include all disorders concerned with the trachea, bronchi, lungs, and pleura. The type, location, and dimension of the process all can lead to more or less marked damage to breathing- related functions.

Mild: Respiratory insufficiency which is hardly noticeable. The breathing test is normal without hypoxic signs. The main symptoms are coughing, mild fever, mild shortage of breath due to fleeting ventilation disturbances caused by mucus formation, and/or pain.

Moderate: Higher-grade respiratory insufficiency characterized by functional dyspnea upon exertion and resulting restriction. A breathing test may still be normal. In addition, record infections with fever which have led to a lowering of general health.

Severe: Marked respiratory insufficiency. Breathing test is failed or is very unsatisfactory. Marked curtailment of performance or activity through hypoxia, infections with high fever, resting dyspnea, and/or demonstrable cyanosis.

Note: All malignant processes of the lungs are rated "severe" and, at the same time, entered under "Chronic Consumptive Processes" (Item 20).

Gastrointestinal Disorders

All disorders which hamper ingestion, digestion, or elimination. Included here are disorders of the esophagus, stomach, intestines, pancreas, gallbladder, and liver as well as disturbances of mastication resulting from impairment of chewing and/or damage to the food transport mechanism.

Mild: Disorders which remain localized in their effect and do not lead to marked functional loss, i.e., the organism is perfectly able to compensate for the disorder.

Moderate: Disorders that impair the functions of one or more organs so that adaptation is limited and only extra demand will lead to distinct functional loss.

Severe: The afflicted organs are so markedly damaged that the functional loss can no longer be compensated. The disorder can affect related tissues and organs and/or have a considerable effect on the total organism, e.g., cachexia.

Note: All malignant processes are rated "severe."

7. Hypersalivation: A report by the patient of excessive and persistent salivary flow and/or frequent swallowing of accumulated saliva which does not substantially impair functioning is rated "mild." When the patient is clearly disturbed by drooling or if the bed pillow is soaked with saliva in the morning, rate "severe." (AMDP-III, 110)

8. Dry Mouth: If the patient notices persistent dryness of the mouth, but is not hampered by it, rate "mild." If speech is affected, rate "moderate." If remedial medication, e.g., lozenges, is necessary, rate "severe." (AMDP-III, 111).

9. Nausea: Slight stomach discomfort is rated "mild"; imminent vomiting ("heaving") is rated "severe." (AMDP-III, 112)

10. Constipation: When bowel movements are not daily, but a laxative is not necessary, rate "mild." A need for a laxative is rated "moderate." If an enema is required, rate "severe." (AMDP-III, 115)

11. Diarrhea: More than one bowel movement per day is rated "mild." If the patient's functioning is disrupted, rate "severe." (AMDP-III, 110)

12. Other: Specify and rate all disorders not subsumed by previous items.

Urogenital Disorders

Chronic renal insufficiency as well as other disorders of the associated urinary system are recorded here.

13. Renal Insufficiency

Mild: Insufficiency with mildly reduced concentration capacity and a negligible increase of creatinine/urea (still within normal limits).

Moderate: Creatinine/urea increased above normal limits under a normal diet; a significant reduction of concentration.

Severe: Decompensated insufficiency with elevated creatinine/N-residue/urea; metabolic acidosis (uremia).

Also record findings under "Chronic Consumptive Processes."

14. Micturition Disturbances: Every impediment to urinating of whatever type should be recorded.

15. Other: Specify and rate any disorders not subsumed in the previous items.

Skeletomuscular Disorders

16. Skeletomuscular Disorders: Include fractures, arthropathies, as well as disorders of the spinal column and other skeletomuscular disorders, e.g., myopathy, myosites. Rating is based on clinical evaluation.

Metabolic Disorders

17. Diabetes Mellitus:

Mild: Fasting blood sugar (FBS) continually or intermittently slightly elevated; pathological glucose tolerance; no glycosuria.

Moderate: Permanently elevated FBS; glycosuria; no secondary organic complications.

Severe: Secondary organic complications, e.g., diabetic angiopathy, eyeground changes, diabetic nephropathy, gangrene, or furunculosis.

18. Other: Specify and rate any other metabolic disorders.

Chronic Pain

19. Chronic Pain: Include all constant or chronically intermittent pain regardless of its etiology and/or demonstrable organic basis. Rating is based on the degree to which the patient feels incapacitated.

Chronic Consumptive Processes

20. Chronic Consumptive Processes: Include all disease processes which are characterized by irreversible progression and lead to progressive physical deterioration. Malignant forms of all disease processes which lead to advanced physical deterioration are recorded, e.g., arteriosclerosis, renal insufficiency, diabetes, tuberculosis. Such encoding overlaps, on the one hand, with previously encoded special organ systems and, on the other hand, with the encoding of the global of health. Such duplication in rating, however, makes possible a differentiation between acute and chronic disease processes – at least globally. The rating of "mild," "moderate," or "severe" is based only on clinical impression.

Other Somatic Disorders

All somatic disorders not included under previous rubics are included here.

21. Blurred Vision: Loss or impairment of accommodation. "Mild" is rated when the patient is aware of blurred vision but is not hampered by it. "Moderate" is rated when reading is impaired. When handwork or reading is no longer possible, rate "severe." (AMDP-III, 121)

22. Increased Perspiration: Not environmentally induced. If a marked tendency toward excessive sweating hinders the patient in his work or is embarrassing in social situations, rate "severe." (AMDP-III, 122)

23. Chills: Complaints of feeling "cold" are rated "mild." Shivering, "goose bumps," or chattering teeth which are independent of the external temperature are rated "severe." (AMDP-III, 130)

24. Excessive Thirst: Frequent or continuous desire to drink. Intake greater than two liters/day or a change in the patient's usual life-style because of a drinking compulsion (as in diabetes insipidus) is rated "severe." Excessive intake due to external heat, i.e., summer weather, is not rated here. (AMDP-III, 108)

25. Reduced Thirst: The patient spontaneously or, upon inquiry, admits to a significantly reduced intake of fluids from premorbid levels. Rate "mild" if this is the only ascertainable symptom. If the reduced thirst leads to exsiccosis (dehydration), rate "severe."

26. Excessive Appetite: "Mild" or "moderate" is rated when the patients eats snacks between meals. "Severe" is rated when there is a significant weight gain or when the patient overeats, i.e., compulsive eating, ravenous appetite, polyphagia, bulimia. (AMDP-III, 107)

27. Decreased Appetite: In comparison with the premorbid norm there is a diminished food intake and/or desire to eat. If the food intake is reduced but is nevertheless sufficient, rate "mild." If it is necessary to urge the patient to eat or he must force himself to eat, rate "moderate." If there is significant weight loss or a complete refusal to eat (anorexia), rate "severe." (AMDP-III, 106)

28. Headache: Every type of headache is included. The rating should be judged by the degree of debility or impairment which the patient experiences as a consequence.

29. Dizziness: All forms of dizziness are rated here – from mild disturbances of orthostatic regulation to severe orthostatic collapse. Frequently described as "faintness or weakness upon rising." (AMDP-III, 118)

30. Other: Specify and rate any other somatic disorders.

Neurological Disorders

When encoding an existing sign under this rubric, the lateralization of the neurological sign – if present – should be noted. If lateralization is absent, encode "BO" (both sides). When lateralization either as a right- or left-sided accentuation (stress) or as a right/left one-sided symptom is present, encode either "LT" (left side) or "RT" (right side). If no neurological disorders of any type are present, circle "O" and proceed to Item 76 ("Handedness").

Olfactory Disorders

31. Olfactory Disorders: Often accompanied by taste disorders. To examine, block one nostril and present aromatic substances to the other. Irritation of the mucous membrane by substances such as vinegar and ammonia can be precipitated in anosmia via the trigeminal nerve; accordingly, those substances should not be used in the olfactory tests.

Visual and Ocular Disorders

32, 33. Central/Peripheral Visual Disorders: Central (visual field) and peripheral (acuity) disturbances should be tested by examining the perimeters of the visual field with the finger and acuity with a standard eye chart. The encoding of right/left differences refers here to the right or left visual field.

34. Central (Lateral) Gaze Paresis: Damage in the system evidenced by arbitrary and ratcheting, sideward ocular movements resulting from cortical and pontine lesions. The rare, vertical ocular paresis is not included here.

35. Oculomotor Paresis: The encoding of right/left differences refers here to the side of the ocular paralysis. A more precise differentiation is not required.

36. Optokinetic Nystagmus: Only encode unceasing nystagmus upon ocular movement or due to bulbar dysfunction.

37. Spontaneous Nystagmus: Only recorded when, with the eyes in normal position, nystagmus is seen with the Frenzel glass – no provocation method.

Hearing Disorders

38, 39. Middle/Inner Ear Disorders: Binaural and monaural hearing should be tested with conversational and whispered speech at a distance of approximately 6 m. Differentiation between middle and inner ear disorders should be tested with a tuning fork in the usual manner. (Rinne and Weber)

Central Motor Disorders

40. Hemiparesis: Unilateral paralysis

41. Paraparesis: Paralysis affecting the lower limbs

42. Quadriparesis: Paralysis affecting the four limbs
Included are centrally incurred pareses with increased muscle tonus and spastic symptoms subdivided into the three most important syndromes: hemiparesis, paraparesis, and quadriparesis. To test for pyramidal symptoms, use the methods of Babinski, Gordon, and Oppenheim.

Central Sensory Disorders

43. Hemihypesthesia

44. Transverse Hypesthesia: Only a gross differentiation between hemi- and transverse hypesthesia is required. Though not individually noted here, all sense qualities should be tested; i.e., touch, pain, temperature, vibration, and kinesthesia.

Peripheral Motor Disorders

45. Distal Motor Disorders

46. Proximal Motor Disorders: Include peripheral, flaccid paralyses with extinct righting reflexes as well as their predominant localization.

Peripheral Sensory Disorders

47. Peripheral Sensory Disorders: Polyneuropathies with their visually distal distribution are differentiated here from other peripheral nerve lesions.

Spinal Cord Lesions (Root Compression Syndromes)

48. Cervical

49. Thoracic

50. Sacrolumbar: All segmented motor and sensory disorders in the cervical, thoracic, and sacrolumbar regions should be included.

Extrapyramidal Disorders

51. Rigidity: Includes increased extrapyramidal tonus with symmetrical resistance to passive movement and, frequently, jerk-like increased tonus (cogwheeling).

52. Moderate/Gross Tremor: These forms of tremor often affect the lower extremities. Determination is based on the rhythmic or arrhythmic movements which are seen "at rest" and as a continuous tremor and which have higher amplitudes than those seen in fine tremor. Parkinsonian tremor is characterized by a frequency of 4–7 beats/s and by "pill rolling."

53. Fine Tremor: This form of tremor is seen frequently in the hands and is recognized by its rhythmic or arrhythmic trembling characterized by small amplitude and rapid frequency. As a rule, it is seen at rest and as a continuous tremor.

54. Akinesia: Absence of automatic movements accompanying walking. Accompanied, as a rule, by a stiff, facial expression and reduced blinking and micrographia. Intentional turning of the head is often accompanied by rotating of the head and upper body "en masse."

55. Akathisia: Irrepressible urge toward movement either through extreme constant and restless "rushing around," inability to sit and/or lie down, or automatic movements such as moving in place while standing, imitative movements, or constant restlessness in the fingers and hands. The restlessness is experienced by the patient as distress.
Dyskinesia: Predominantly pharmacogenic but also includes dysfunctional, spasmodic movements on the basis of atrophic cerebral processes.

56. Acute Dyskinesia: Transient dyskinesia appears most frequently in the so-called "bucco-linguo-oral dyskinesia", e.g., under treatment with neuroleptics in which there is a spasm-like tonic innervation of the tongue, mouth, floor of the mouth, nape, neck, and cervical musculature. Can also be accompanied by torticollis, torso spasm, and similar dystonic movements.

57. Tardive (Persistent) Dyskinesia: Without regard to the separately cited akathisia (Item 55), include all other persistent disorders of movement of the extrapyramidal type, e.g., constant perioral unrest (mumbling), tongue rolling. Tics are included under "Other CNS Disorders" and stereotypy under "Psychomotor Disorders." In case of doubt, the assignment should be to the rubric of highest probable etiology.

Disorders of Coordination

58. Intention Tremor: The tremor begins at the initiation of voluntary movement.

59. Pointing Ataxia: Difficulty in pointing to nose with finger, etc.

60. Postural Ataxia: Difficulty in maintaining stance.

61. Gait Ataxia: Difficulty with gait. Confirmed by testing along usual neurological lines. The encoding of left (LT) or right (RT) is determined by the predominant deviation from normal orientation. Unsystematized deviations are scored "BO" (both).

Primitive Reflexes

Primitive motor patterns which can be observed in healthy babies and in adults as a result of disintegrating cerebral processes. They can appear both spontaneously and as evoked reflexes. They are, therefore not reflexes in the usual sense. An entry is made if at least one of the three following, defined reflexes is present.

62. Perioral (Sucking) Reflex: Record if sucking movements are evoked by touching the mouth or if, after touching the lips, the head turns in the direction of the touching object. In the early stages of illness, this effect can be evoked through an optical stimulus.

63. Grasp Reflex: Involuntary grasping when the palm of hand is stimulated by touch. Groping: The patient's hand continues to "grope" after the slowly retreating stimulus.

64. Palmomental Reflex: By stimulating the inner palm in the region of the ball of the thumb, e.g., with a vibrating tuning fork, a quick, short contraction of the musculus mentalis on the same side is evoked.

65. Other: Specify and rate any other pathological findings, e.g., orbicularis-occuli reflex.

Equilibrium Disorders

66. Equilibrium Disorders: Encode any disorders of equilibrium and note the direction of disequilibrium.

Bulbar Disorders

Disorders of the brain stem which are usually observed as slurring of speech and/or difficulties in swallowing.

67. Speech Disorders: Heavy, slurred speech.

68. Swallowing: Dysphagia.

Cerebral Seizures

All forms of cerebral seizure are to be included. Most forms exhibit seizure-like, transient disturbances of consciousness in which, as a rule, motor and/or sensory and autonomic phenomena emerge. The symptoms, in every case, are expressions of a functional cerebral disorder.

69. Generalized Primary Epilepsy: Mainly paroxysms of the general type are to be recorded here. Grand mal status epilepticus is included.

70. Generalized Secondary Epilepsy: Here the decision should be made from clinical observation and not on the basis of EEG findings. Also documented are episodes which begin as one of the focal seizures named above and then evolve into a grand mal seizure.

71. Partial (Focal) Epilepsy: All focal seizures belong here, e.g., motoric and sensory Jacksonian seizures, adversive seizures. The focus is based on clinical symptomatology, not on the EEG.

72. Unclassified Epilepsy: All syndromes usually subsumed under epilepsy, e.g., myoclonic epilepsy and epilepsia partialis continua (Kojewnikoff's epilepsy), are documented here. This item may also be used when the examiner is not clear as to which form of epilepsy is present.

Other CNS Disorders

Here the examiner can specify and rate disorders which do not fit under any previous rubric.

73. Peripheral Disorders

74. Central Disorders

75. Psychogenic Disorders

Handedness

76. Handedness: Can be determined globally or with the rating scale described below. Handedness (skill) can be recorded as an indirect indicator of hemisphere dominance which at present cannot be ascertained with certainty. Since it is assumed on the basis of previous investigations that there is no general hemisphere dominance, but rather varying dominance for specific functions, handedness is by far the most invetigated and the easiest skill to ascertain clinically and can therefore be used to document dominance. The present assessment is restricted to this approach.

By handedness is meant the preference for one hand over the other to perform specific activities, e.g., writing, opening doors, ball throwing, pointing, combing, hammering. The assessment of handedness is not entirely dependent upon the chosen test method. Unequivocal assignment to one hemisphere can be made only if hemiparesis and simultaneous speech disturbance point to the "dominant" hemisphere.

The evaluation of handedness is based either on the clinical observation of the motor processes, particularly in writing, or upon the following modified test of Nutzhorn and Suchenwirt. The test consists of the following seven simple tasks which are carried out in pantomine:

1. Drawing a circle in the air
2. Sharpening a pencil
3. Hammering
4. Striking a match
5. Combing hair
6. Shining shoes
7. Brushing teeth

Two points are scored for completing each subtest with the right hand; zero points for preference of the left hand. If the patient uses the right hand one time and the left hand another time, or if he shows a definite uncertainty about the preferred hand or uses both hands, score 1 point. This will produce a range of scores between 14 points for completing all tasks with the right hand and zero points for successfully accomplishing all tasks with the left hand. To determine handedness, the range is divided into three levels:

0– 4 points = Left handedness
5– 9 points = Ambidexterity
10–14 points = Right handedness

Part 6 – Diagnoses

Three psychiatric and four physical diagnoses may be entered in this section. While the WHO International Classification of Diseases (ICD-9) is the system of diagnosis used exclusively in the German AGP, investigators in the United States may prefer to use the DSM-III for psychiatric diagnosis. An item to designate the choice of system has been added to this version of the AGP.

Status

For partial and 24-hour hospitalized patients, a final diagnosis should be made. For outpatients, the diagnosis made at the time of the examination should be encoded.

Clinical Experience

One entry only. Refers to the number of years of clinical psychiatric experience possessed by the examiner.

$>$ *1 yr:* Less than one year
1–3 yr: One to less than 3 years
3–5 yr: Three to less than 5 years
$>$ *5 yr:* Five years or more

Psychiatric Diagnoses

First check whether ICD-9 or DSM-III is employed for psychiatric diagnoses. Use the same system for all psychiatric diagnoses.

Example: ICD-9 ____ DSM-III _✓_

A maximum of three psychiatric diagnoses may be encoded. When several diagnoses are made, the first diagnosis should reflect the illness which most characterizes the clinical picture. For each diagnosis made, six entries are required:

1, 2. Name/Code: The name and code number of the diagnosis should be stated in the exact terms of the diagnostic system employed.

Example: Not "depressive episode," rather "Major affective disorders recurrent"

Most ICD-9 and DSM-III diagnoses require a minimum of four digits – a fifth digit may also be used in DSM-III. To defer diagnosis, write "Deferred" and enter the appropriate number for "Deferred Diagnosis." While both name and number are equally important, name is à la Orwell "more equal" and must always be encoded. Lastly, write legibly!

3. ICD-9 Diagnostic Section: Applies only to ICD-9; may be left blank with DSM-III. Some ICD-9 codes are alphanumeric, i.e., contain a letter as well as numbers. When using such codes, check the appropriate letter code and then encode the required digits.

E = Section XVII, Accidents, Poisoning, and Violence (External Causes)
N = Section II, Neoplasms
Y = Section XVII, Special Conditions and Examinations without illness

4. Diagnostic Certitude: One entry only. The examiner's degree of confidence, i.e., certainty, in the aforenamed diagnosis. The degrees are:

MI: Minimal or low degree of certitude
MO: Moderate or average degree of certitude
HI: High degree of certitude. "You'd bet on it."

5. Age at First Manifestation: Refers to the first appearance of the aforementioned illness. The age intervals are given in decades except for the first interval, which encompasses the first two decades of life.

6. Certitude (Age): Refers to examiner's degree of confidence (certainty) in the aforenamed age interval.
This procedure is followed for each psychiatric diagnosis. If only one psychiatric diagnosis is made, leave the two remaining encoding areas blank.

Somatic (Physical) Diagnoses

These diagnoses are all encoded in the ICD-9 system. A maximum of four diagnoses may be encoded. If no somatic diagnoses are made, check "None" and leave remaining areas blank. The instructions for encoding this section are the same as those give for psychiatric diagnoses.

Appendix A: German and English Lists of Psychopathological Symptoms[1]

German	English
Bewußtseinsstörungen	*Disorders of Consciousness*
1. Bewußtseinsverminderung	1. Lowered vigilance (1)
2. Bewußtseinseinengung	2. Narrowed consciousness (3)
3. Bewußtseinstrübung	3. Clouded consciousness
4. Hypnagoge Zustände	4. Hypnagogic states
5. Parasomnische Bewußtseinseinlage	5. Parasomnia
Orientierungsstörungen	*Disturbances of Orientation*
6. Zeitlich	6. Time (5)
7. Örtlich	7. Place (6)
8. Situativ	8. Situation (7)
9. Autopsychisch	9. Self (8)
Aufmerksamkeits- und Gedächtnisstörungen	*Disorders of Attention and Memory*
10. Auffassungsstörungen	10. Apperception (10)
11. Konzentrationsstörungen	11. Concentration (11)
12. Merkfähigkeitsstörungen	12. Memorization (12)

[1] AMDP-III item numbers are given in parentheses

German	English
13. Merkfähigkeitsstörungen für Zahlen	13. Memorization for numbers
14. Merkfähigkeitsstörungen für Wörter	14. Memorization for words
15. Merkfähigkeitsstörungen für Gegenstände	15. Memorization for objects
16. Merkfähigkeitsstörungen für Formen	16. Memorization for forms
17. Merkfähigkeitsstörungen für Personen	17. Memorization for people
18. Merkfähigkeitsstörungen für Farben	18. Memorization for colors
19. Störung des Frischgedächtnisses	19. Recent memory
20. Störung des Altgedächtnisses	20. Remote memory
21. Zeitgitterstörungen	21. Forgetfulness
22. Gesteigerte Löschvorgänge	22. Ecmnesia
23. Hypermnesie des Altgedächtnisses	23. Hypermnesia (remote memory)
24. Konfabulationen	24. Confabulation (13)
25. Paramnesien	25. Paramnesias (14)
26. Suggestibilität/Induzierbarkeit	26. Suggestibility
Formale Denkstörungen	*Formal Disturbances of Thinking*
27. Gehemmt	27. Inhibited (experienced) (15)
28. Verlangsamt	28. Retarded (observed) (16)
29. Umständlich	29. Circumstantial (17)

German	English
30. Eingeengt	30. Restricted (18)
31. Perseverierend	31. Perseveration (19)
32. Grübeln	32. Rumination (20)
33. Gedankendrängen	33. Pressured (21)
34. Ideenflüchtig	34. Flight of ideas (22)
35. Vorbeireden	35. Tangential (23)
36. Gesperrt/Gedankenabreißen	36. Blocking (24)
37. Inkohärent/zerfahren	37. Incoherence (25)
38. Neologismen	38. Neologisms (26)
39. Beschleunigt	39. Accelerated thinking (P3)
40. Störung des Abstraktionsvermögens	40. Impaired abstraction
41. Störung des Kombinatorischen Denkens	41. Conceptual impairment
42. Störung der Kritikfähigkeit	42. Impaired judgment
Befürchtungen, Zwänge, Phobien	*Fears, Compulsions, Phobias*
43. Mißstrauen	43. Suspiciousness (27)
44. Hypochondrie	44. Hypochondriasis (28)
45. Phobien	45. Phobias (29)
46. Zwangsdenken	46. Obsessive thoughts (30)
47. Zwangsimpulse	47. Compulsive impulses (31)
48. Zwangshandlungen	48. Compulsive actions (32)
Wahn	*Delusions*
49. Wahnstimmung	49. Delusional mood (33)

German	English
50. Wahnwahrnehmung	50. Delusional perceptions (34)
51. Wahneinfall	51. Sudden delusional thoughts (35)
52. Wahngedanken	52. Delusional ideas (36)
53. Systematisierter Wahn	53. Systematized delusions (37)
54. Wahndynamik	54. Delusional dynamics (38)
55. Beziehungswahn	55. Delusions of reference (39)
56. Beeinträchtigungswahn	56. Delusions of persecution (40)
57. Eifersuchtswahn	57. Delusions of jealousy (41)
58. Schuldwahn	58. Delusions of guilt (42)
59. Verarmungswahn	59. Delusions of impoverishment (43)
60. Hypochondrischer Wahn	60. Hypochondriacal delusions (44)
61. Größenwahn	61. Delusions of grandeur (45)
62. Andere Wahninhalte	62. Other delusions (46)
Sinnestäuschungen	*Disorders of Perception*
63. Illusionen	63. Illusions (47)
64. Stimmenhören	64. Verbal hallucinations (48)
65. Andere akustische Halluzinationen	65. Other auditory hallucinations (49)
66. Optische Halluzinationen	66. Visual hallucinations (50)
67. Körperhalluzinationen	67. Bodily hallucinations (51)

German	English
68. Geruchs-Geschmackshalluzinationen	68. Olfactory/gustatory hallucinations (52)
Ich-Störungen	*Disorders of EGO*
69. Derealisation	69. Derealization (53)
70. Depersonalisation	70. Depersonalization (54)
71. Gedankenausbreitung	71. Thought broadcasting (55)
72. Gedankenentzug	72. Thought withdrawal (56)
73. Gedankeneingebung	73. Thought insertion (57)
74. Andere Fremdbeeinflussungserlebnisse	74. Other feelings of alien influence
Störungen der Affektivität	*Disorders of Affect*
75. Ratlos	75. Perplexity (59)
76. Gefühl der Gefühlslosigkeit	76. Feelings of loss of feeling (60)
77. Affektarm (einschl. Anhedonie)	77. Blunted affect (61)
78. Störung der Vitalgefühle	78. Loss of vitality (62)
79. Deprimiert	79. Depressed mood (63)
80. Hoffnungslos	80. Hopelessness (64)
81. Ängstlich	81. Anxiety (65)
82. Euphorisch	82. Euphoria (66)
83. Dysphorisch	83. Dysphoria (67)
84. Gereizt (einschl. gespannt)	84. Irritability (68)
85. Innerlich unruhig	85. Inner restlessness (69)
86. Klagsam/jammerig	86. Complaintativeness (70)
87. Insuffizienzgefühle	87. Feelings of inadequacy (71)

German	English
88. Gesteigerte Selbstwertgefühle	88. Exaggerated self-esteem (72)
89. Schuldgefühle	89. Feelings of guilt (73)
90. Verarmungsgefühle	90. Feelings of impoverishment (74)
91. Ambivalent	91. Ambivalence (75)
92. Parathymie	92. Parathymia (76)
93. Affektlabil	93. Affective lability (77)
94. Affektinkontinent	94. Affective incontinence (78)
95. Affektstarr	95. Affective rigidity (79)
Antriebs- und Psychomotor.-Störungen	*Disturb. of Drive and Psychomotility*
96. Antriebsarm	96. Lack of drive (80)
97. Antriebsgehemmt	97. Inhibition of drive (81)
98. Stuporos	98. Stuporous
99. Antriebsgesteigert	99. Increased drive (82)
100. Motorisch unruhig	100. Motor restlessness (83)
101. Parakinese	101. Parakinesia (84)
102. Manieriert, bizarres Verhalten	102. Mannerisms (85)
103. Theatralisch	103. Histrionics (86)
104. Mutistisch	104. Mutism (87)
105. Logorrhoisch	105. Logorrhea (88)
106. Negativistisch	106. Negativism
107. Entschlußunfähig	107. Indecisiveness
108. Psychoorganisches Syndrom	108. Psychoorganic Syndrome

German	English
Werkzeugstörungen Global	*Global Performance Disturbances*
109. Aphasien	109. Aphasia
110. Agnosien	110. Agnosia
111. Apraxien	111. Apraxia
Fronto-parietale Störungen	*Frontoparietal Disturbances*
112. Frontale Apraxie	112. Frontal apraxia
113. Gesichtsapraxie	113. Facial apraxia
114. Hochfrontales Antriebssyndrom	114. Prefrontal impulse syndrome
115. Fronto-basales Antriebssyndrom	115. Frontobasal impulse syndrome
116. Motorische Aphasie	116. Motor aphasia
Occipitale Störungen	*Occipital Disturbances*
117. Störungen des Farbempfindens/Erkennen	117. Color perception/ recognizing
118. Störungen des Farbempfindens/Benennen	118. Color perception/ naming
119. Störungen des Farbempfindens/Vorstellen	119. Color perception/ visualizing
120. Visuelle Agnosie	120. Visual agnosia
121. Prosopagnosie	121. Prosopagnosia
122. Dysmorphopsie	122. Dysmorphopsia

German	English
Parieto-occipitale Störungen	*Parieto-occipital Disturbances*
123. Stereoagnosie	123. Stereoagnosia
124. Somatotopagnosie	124. Somatagnosia
125. Anosognosie	125. Anosognosia
126. Nachsprechaphasie	126. Conduction aphasia
127. Alexie	127. Alexia
128. Agraphie	128. Agraphia
129. Akalkulie	129. Acalculia
130. Ideokinetische Apraxie	130. Ideomotor apraxia
131. Ideatorische Apraxie	131. Ideational apraxia
132. Konstruktive Apraxie	132. Constructional apraxia
Temporale Störungen	*Temporal Lobe Disorders*
133. Amnestische Aphasie	133. Amnestic aphasia
134. Sensorische Aphasie	134. Sensory aphasia
Circadiane Besonderheiten	*Circadian Disturbances*
135. Morgens schlechter	135. Worse in AM (89)
136. Abends schlechter	136. Worse in PM (90)
137. Abends besser	137. Better in PM (91)
138. Nächtl. Exazerbationen	138. Nighttime exacerbations
139. Alternier	139. Symptom alternation
Schlaf- und Vigilanzstörungen	*Sleep and Vigilance Disturbances*
140. Einschlafstörungen	140. Difficulty falling asleep (101)

German	English
141. Durchschlafstörungen	141. Interrupted sleep (102)
142. Früherwachen	142. Early waking
143. Schlafdauer verlängert	143. Prolonged sleep
144. Schlafdauer verkürzt	144. Shortened sleep (103)
145. Nächtliche Unruhe	145. Nighttime restlessness
146. Nächtliche Verwirrtheitszustände	146. Nighttime confusional state
147. Schläfrigkeit Tagsüber	147. Drowsiness (daytime) (105)
148. Umkehrung des Tag-Nacht Rhythmus	148. Day-night rhythm reversal
149. Gesteigerte Traumtätigkeit	149. Increased dreaming
Störungen des Sozialverhaltens	*Disturbances of Social Behavior*
150. Sozialer Rückzug	150. Social withdrawal (92)
151. Soziale Umtriebigkeit	151. Excessive social contact (93)
152. Aggressivität	152. Aggressiveness (94)
153. Suizidalität	153. Suicidal tendencies (95)
154. Selbstbeschädigung	154. Self-mutilation (96)
155. Mangel an Krankheitsgefühl	155. Lack of feeling (97)
156. Mangel an Krankheitseinsicht	156. Lack of insight (98)
157. Ablehnung der Behandlung	157. Uncooperativeness (99)
158. Dissimulationstendenz	158. Dissimulation
159. Verwahrlosung	159. Self-neglect
160. Nahrungsablehnung	160. Refusal of nourishment
161. Sexualität vermindert	161. Decreased libido (109)
162. Sexualität gesteigert	162. Increased libido (P 5)

German	English
Hilfs- und Pflegebedürftigkeit	*Social and Nursing Needs*
163. Bei finanziellen Angelegenheiten	163. Financial needs
164. Im Haushalt	164. Housekeeping
165. Versorgung mit Medizin und ärztliche Betreuung	165. Medical care
166. Gehen	166. Walking
167. Sich ankleiden	167. Dressing self
168. Sich waschen	168. Personal hygiene
169. Essen	169. Eating
170. Sich beschäftigen	170. Leisure activities
171. Benutzen von öffentlichen Verkehrsmitteln	171. Transportation
172. Kaustörungen	172. Chewing
173. Bettlägerigkeit	173. Bedridden
174. Incontinentia urinae	174. Urinary incontinence
175. Incontinentia alvi	175. Fecal incontinence
176. Beschmiert sich und Umgebung	176. Smearing
Befundunsicherheit	*Reliability of Information*
Zusatzuntersuchungen	*Additional Examinations*
EKG	EKG
EEG	EEG
Echoenzephalogramm	Echoencephalography
CT	CAT scan
Szintigramm	Scintiscan
Dopplersonogramm	Doppler sonography
Angiogramm	Angiography

German	English
Elektronystagmogramm (ENG)	Electronystagmography
Lumbalpunktion (LP)	Lumbar puncture
Pneumenzephalogramm (PEG)	Pneumoencephalog-raphy
Elektromyogramm (EMG)	Electromyography
Psychologische Tests	Psychological tests
r. CBF	Regional cerebral blood flow
andere	Other

Appendix B: German and English Lists of Somatic Signs[1]

German	English
1. Körperlicher Gesundheitszustand (global)	1. Global State of Health
Allgemeine körperliche Störungen	*General Somatic Disturbances*
Kardiovaskuläre Störungen	*Cardiovascular Disturbances*
2. Herzinsuffizienz	2. Cardiac insufficiency
3. Herzrhythmusstörungen	3. Dysrhythmia
4. Hypertonie	4. Hypertension
5. Andere	5. Other
6. *Erkrankungen des respiratorischen Systems*	6. *Respiratory Disorders*
Erkrankungen des Verdauungssystems	*Gastrointestinal Disorders*
7. Hypersalivation	7. Hypersalivation (110)
8. Mundtrockenheit	8. Dry mouth (111)
9. Übelkeit	9. Nausea (112)
10. Obstipation	10. Constipation (115)
11. Diarrhoe	11. Diarrhea (116)
12. Andere	12. Other

[1] AMDP-III item numbers are given in parentheses

German	English
Erkrankungen des Urogenitalsystems	*Urogenital Disturbances*
13. Niereninsuffizienz	13. Renal insufficiency
14. Miktionsstörungen	14. Micturition disturbances
15. Andere	15. Other
16. Erkrankungen des Bewegungsapparates	16. *Skeletomuscular disturbances*
Stoffwechselstörungen	*Metabolic Disturbances*
17. Diabetes Mellitus	17. Diabetes mellitus
18. Andere	18. Other
19. *Chronische Schmerzzustände*	19. *Chronic Pain*
20. *Chronische konsumptive Prozesse*	*20. Chronic Consumptive Processes*
Sonstige körperliche Störungen	*Other Somatic Disorders*
21. Akkomodationsstörungen	21. Blurred vision (121)
22. Schwitzen vermehrt	22. Excessive perspiration (122)
23. Frösteln	23. Chills (123)
24. Durst vermehrt	24. Excessive thirst (108)
25. Durst vermindert	25. Reduced thirst
26. Appetit vermehrt	26. Excessive appetite (107)
27. Appetit vermindert	27. Decreased appetite (106)
28. Kopfschmerzen	28. Headache (126)
29. Schwindel	29. Dizziness (118)
30. Andere	30. Other

German	English
Neurologische Störungen	*Neurological Disorders*
31. *Geruchsstörungen*	31. Olfactory Disorders
Seh- und Blickstörungen	*Visual and Ocular Disorders*
32. Zentrale Sehstörungen	32. Central visual disturbance
33. Periphere Sehstörungen	33. Peripheral visual disturbance
34. Zentrale Blickparese	34. Central gaze paresis
35. Augenmuskelparese	35. Oculomotor paresis
36. Blickrichtungsnystagmus	36. Optokinetic nystagmus
37. Spontannystagmus	37. Spontaneous nystagmus
Hörstörungen	*Hearing Disorders*
38. Mittelohr	38. Middle ear
39. Innenohr	39. Inner ear
Zentrale motorische Störungen	*Central Motor Disorders*
40. Hemiparese	40. Hemiparesis
41. Paraparese	41. Paraparesis
42. Tetraparese	42. Quadriparesis
Zentrale Sensibilitätsstörungen	*Central Sensory Disorders*
43. Hemihypaesthesie	43. Hemihypesthesia
44. Querschnitt	44. Transverse hypesthesia

German	English
Periphere motorische Störungen	*Peripheral Motor Disorders*
45. Distal	45. Distal
46. Proximal	46. Proximal
47. *Periphere Sensibilitätsstörungen*	47. Peripheral Sensory Disorders
Radikuläre Läsion	*Spinal Cord Lesions*
48. Zervikal	48. Cervical
49. Thorakal	49. Thoracic
50. Lumbosakral	50. Sacrolumbar
Extrapyramidale Motorik	*Extrapyramidal Disorders*
51. Rigor	51. Rigidity
52. Tremor grobschlägig	52. Gross tremor
53. Tremor feinschlägig	53. Fine tremor
54. Akinese	54. Akinesia
55. Akathisie	55. Akathisia
56. Akute Dyskinesen	56. Acute dyskinesia
57. Persistierende Dyskinesen	57. Tardive dyskinesia
Koordinationsstörungen	*Disorders of Coordination*
58. Intentionstremor	58. Intention tremor
59. Zeigeataxie	59. Pointing ataxia
60. Standataxie	60. Postural ataxia
61. Gangataxie	61. Gait ataxia

German	English
Primitivreflexe	*Primitive Reflexes*
62. Perioral	62. Perioral reflex
63. Greifreflex	63. Grasp reflex
64. Palmomentalreflex	64. Palmomental reflex
65. Andere	65. Other
66. *Gleichgewichtsstörungen*	66. *Equilibrium Disorders*
Bulbäre Symptome	*Bulbar Disorders*
67. Sprechen	67. Speaking
68. Schlucken	68. Swallowing
Cerebrale Anfälle	*Cerebral Seizures*
69. Generalisierte primäre Epilepsie	69. Generalized primary epilepsy
70. Generalisierte sekundäre Epilepsie	70. Generalized secondary epilepsy
71. Partielle (lokale) Epilepsie	71. Focal epilepsy
72. Unklassifizierte Epilepsie	72. Unclassified epilepsy
Sonstige Störungen d. ZNS	*Other CNS Disorders*
73. Peripher	73. Peripheral
74. Zentral	74. Central
75. Psychogen	75. Psychogenic
76. *Händigkeit*	76. *Handedness*

References

The extensive bibliography contained in *The AMDP System: Manual for the Assessment and Documentation of Psychopathology* (6) provides background for much of the material contained in this volume. All titles listed below are rendered in English. The original language of the articles is denoted by: G = German, F = French, E = English, S = Spanish.

1. Association for Gerontopsychiatry (1973) Ciompi L, Kanowski S (eds) The AGP System: Manual for the documentation of psychopathology in geriatric patients. Provisional draft. G
2. Ban TA (1978) The AMP System in English. In: Deniker P, Radouco-Thomas C, Villeneuve A (eds) Proceedings Xth Congress CINP. Pergamon Press, London, pp 1575–1579. E
3. Ban TA, Lehmann HE, Galvan L, Pecknold JC, Climan M (1974) A transcultural study with clomacran. Comparison of two assessment methods. Curr Ther Res 16:971–989. E
4. Ban TA, Jamieson RC, Lehmann HE (1978) AMP Psychopathological Assessment Form. Development of the English version. Presented at 13th Annual GWAN Meeting, Ottawa. E
5. Bobon DP, Pichot P (to be published) Videotaped evaluation of the French adaptation of the AMDP Psychopathology Scale. Transcultural vs individual divergence. Actas Luso Esp Neurol Psiquiatr. S
6. Bolm H, Buckler R, Freudenthal K, Kanowski S, Lieberz K, Schroter O, Werner V (1973) Initial experience and findings of a comparative study of different geriatric populations with a gerontopsychiatric documentation system. Janssen Symposien. Gerontopsychiatrie 3, Düsseldorf, pp 161–187. G
7. Busch H, Fahndrich E, Freudenthal K, Renfordt E (1975) On the modifications and further development of the AMP System. Report on a symposium and training seminar. Pharmakopsychiatr Neuropsychopharmakol 8:1970–1975. G
8. Ciompi L (1976) Systems of documentation in psychiatry. The AMP and AGP Systems. Psychol Med 8:441–452. F
9. Ciompi L, Kobrianus A, Müller C (1973) Basic documentation in gerontopsychiatry. The AGP System. Janssen Symposium vol. 13. Janssen, Düsseldorf. G
10. Ciompi L, Lobrinus A, Müller C, Wertheimer J, Frosst N, Helmchen H, Hermann U, Kanowski S (1972) Proposal for a Gerontopsychiatric documentation System. Janssen Symposien. Gerontopsychiatrie 2, Düsseldorf, 211–232. G

11. Frost N, Helmchen H, Hermann U, Kanowski S (1971) Proposal for a symptom catalog for gerontopsychiatric documentation. Janssen Symposien. Gerontopsychiatrie 1, Düsseldorf, 224–254. G
12. Guy W (1976) ECDEU assessment manual for psychopharmacology. DHEW Pub No. (ADM) USGPO. Washington DC, pp 76–338. E
13. Guy W, Ban TA (eds) (1982) The AMDP System: Manual for the assessment and documentation of psychopathology. Springer, Berlin Heidelberg New York. E
14. Hermann U (1972) Possibilities and limits in the documentation of gerontopsychiatric social data. Janssen Symposien. Gerontopsychiatrie 2, Düsseldorf, 233–244. G
15. Jaspers K (1959) General psychopathology (Allgemeine Psychopathologie), 7th edn. Springer, Berlin Heidelberg New York. G
16. Junkers G, Kanowski S, Paur R (1976) Research training and case record maintenance from the view of a division of gerontopsychiatry. Z Gerontologie 9:151–175. G
17. Scharfetter C (1972) The AMP System (Das AMP-System), 2nd edn. Springer, Berlin Heidelberg New York. G
18. von Cranach M, Strauss A (1977) On further development of the AMP System. Report on the 2nd AMP symposium and training seminar. Pharmakopsychiatr Neuropsychopharmakol 10:254–261. G
19. Woggon B, Baumann U, Angst J (1978) Interreliability of AMP symptoms. Arch Psychiatr Nervenkr 225:73–85. G

Index

The first numeric refers to page number. The second letter/numeric, refers to AGP item, i.e., IB = Identification Block, DD = Demographic Data, PH = Psychiatric History, PS = Psychopathological Symptoms, SS = Somatic Signs.

GPSR Compliance

The European Union's (EU) General Product Safety Regulation (GPSR) is a set of rules that requires consumer products to be safe and our obligations to ensure this.

If you have any concerns about our products, you can contact us on ProductSafety@springernature.com

In case Publisher is established outside the EU, the EU authorized representative is:

Springer Nature Customer Service Center GmbH
Europaplatz 3
69115 Heidelberg, Germany

Batch number: 10704701

Printed by Printforce, the Netherlands